Textbook of
**Physiotherapy for Clinical
Cardio-Thoracic Conditions**

Textbook of Physiotherapy for Clinical Cardio-Thoracic Conditions

SECOND EDITION

GB Madhuri
MPT (Orthopedics, Neurology) PGDPC DYT
Physical Therapist
USA

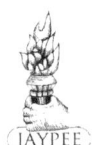

JAYPEE BROTHERS MEDICAL PUBLISHERS
The Health Sciences Publisher
New Delhi | London

Jaypee Brothers Medical Publishers (P) Ltd

Headquarters
Jaypee Brothers Medical Publishers (P) Ltd
EMCA House, 23/23-B
Ansari Road, Daryaganj
New Delhi 110 002, India
Landline: +91-11-23272143, +91-11-23272703
+91-11-23282021, +91-11-23245672
Email: jaypee@jaypeebrothers.com

Corporate Office
Jaypee Brothers Medical Publishers (P) Ltd
4838/24, Ansari Road, Daryaganj
New Delhi 110 002, India
Phone: +91-11-43574357
Fax: +91-11-43574314
Email: jaypee@jaypeebrothers.com

Overseas Office
J.P. Medical Ltd
83 Victoria Street, London
SW1H 0HW (UK)
Phone: +44 20 3170 8910
Fax: +44 (0)20 3008 6180
Email: info@jpmedpub.com

Website: www.jaypeebrothers.com
Website: www.jaypeedigital.com

© 2022, Jaypee Brothers Medical Publishers

The views and opinions expressed in this book are solely those of the original contributor(s)/author(s) and do not necessarily represent those of editor(s) and publisher of the book.

All rights reserved. No part of this publication may be reproduced, stored or transmitted in any form or by any means, electronic, mechanical, photocopying, recording or otherwise, without the prior permission in writing of the publishers/editors.

All brand names and product names used in this book are trade names, service marks, trademarks or registered trademarks of their respective owners. The publisher is not associated with any product or vendor mentioned in this book.

Medical knowledge and practice change constantly. This book is designed to provide accurate, authoritative information about the subject matter in question. However, readers are advised to check the most current information available on procedures included and check information from the manufacturer of each product to be administered, to verify the recommended dose, formula, method and duration of administration, adverse effects and contraindications. It is the responsibility of the practitioner to take all appropriate safety precautions. Neither the publisher nor the author(s)/editor(s) assume any liability for any injury and/or damage to persons or property arising from or related to use of material in this book.

This book is sold on the understanding that the publisher is not engaged in providing professional medical services. If such advice or services are required, the services of a competent medical professional should be sought.

Every effort has been made where necessary to contact holders of copyright to obtain permission to reproduce copyright material. If any have been inadvertently overlooked, the publisher will be pleased to make the necessary arrangements at the first opportunity.

Inquiries for bulk sales may be solicited at: jaypee@jaypeebrothers.com

Textbook of Physiotherapy for Clinical Cardio-Thoracic Conditions

First Edition: 2008

Second Edition: **2022**

ISBN: 978-93-5465-948-5

Dedicated
To my beautiful daughters
Manasvini Santhoshi
and
Juhika Santhoshi

Preface to the Second Edition

Textbook of Physiotherapy for Clinical Cardio-Thoracic Conditions has been design to cater the needs of the students of Bachelor's and Master's degree in Physiotherapy. This book is also useful for physiotherapists, teachers, doctors, rehabilitation professionals, and other paramedics.

This book has been prepared as per the curriculum of Clinical Cardio-Thoracic subject devised as per MCI regulations at various universities in India and abroad. Few of the universities are NTR University of Health Sciences, Andhra Pradesh, Dr MGR Medical University, Chennai, Rajiv Gandhi University of Health Sciences, Bengaluru, Manipal Academy of Higher Education, Manipal and Gujarat University, Gujarat and many more universities both in India and abroad especially preparation guide for NPTE – National Physical Therapy Examination which is Licensure exam for Practice in USA .

This is essential and basic subject of physiotherapy for the undergraduate and as well as postgraduate courses. Very few number of textbooks by foreign authors are available in the market which are suitable for the students and to avoid confusion in understanding each topic of the entire subject and referring many books for topics in the syllabus. Recently lots of advances have taken place in the field of Cardio-Thoracic. Utmost efforts have been made to cover all the necessary aspects of subject. All chapters have been written in a very simple and clearly expressed.

Physiotherapy is an ever advancing field. The recent advances have made in physiotherapy are very interesting and playing an important role in working women and men with regard to ergonomics at work place to prevent further complications like low backache, etc. So maintain fitness, posture, stress-free techniques like relaxation and breathing. All these techniques are found to be effective and important nowadays. Utmost efforts have been made in this book up-to-date from the introduction to the recent advances. All these aspects have been covered with details.

I have tried to give a fairly complete coverage of the subject describing the most common methods known to be employed by physiotherapist at appropriate time. The intension is to explain how these methods work and their effects. I have tried to lay the foundation of the principles of physiotherapy for a thorough understanding of these principles will ultimately lead to safer and more effective lifestyle.

Chapter One: Anatomy in brief about lungs, bronchi, bronchopulmonary segments, relationship of the bony thorax and lungs to each other and to the abdominal contents, variations of the bony cage in conditions like cervical rib, rickets-rachitic rosary, pigeon chest, funnel chest, scoliosis, kyphosis, movements of thorax like bucket handle and pump handle movements. Muscles of respiration involved in inspiration and expiration, anatomy of heart, blood supply, electrical activity of the myocardium and normal ECG.

Chapter Two: Physiology and covers topics like physiological control of respiration, functions of medullary and pontine respiratory centers and central and peripheral chemoreceptors, maintenance of Blood Pressure, cough reflex, mechanical factors involved in breathing and factors affecting lung compliance and airway resistance, diffusion of oxygen and carbon dioxide in the lungs, ventilation, perfusion and their interrelationship, energy expenditure of various common activity of daily living, pulmonary function assessment includes pulmonary function tests, tests performed by physical therapist, assessment of COPD patients, basis and value of the blood gas analysis. Principles of the cardiovascular stress testing, arrhythmia, syncope and its management, fundamentals of ECG, recording and basic interpretation.

Chapter Three: Explains about cardiac surgery for closed heart surgery conditions that includes both congenital heart diseases conditions like patent Ductus Arteriosus and Coarctation of aorta and acquired heart disease conditions like mitral stenosis and aortic stenosis.

Chapter Four: Explains about cardiac surgery conditions especially open heart surgery that includes both congenital conditions like atrial septal defect, ventricular septal defect, pulmonary stenosis, tetralogy of Fallot, transposition of great vessels, AV malformation and acquired conditions like mitral stenosis, mitral regurgitation, aortic stenosis, coronary artery disease, angina pectoris, cardiac failure, congestive heart failure.

Chapter Five: Thoracic surgery conditions like fracture ribs, flail chest, stove in chest, pneumothorax, hemothorax, hemopneumothorax, lung contusion and laceration, injury to heart, great vessels and bronchus, empyema intercostal drainage, rib resection, decortication and window operation pulmonary tuberculosis, Tuberculoma, bronchiectasis sicca, bronchostenosis, massive hemoptysis, empyema, suppurative lesions of lung like bronchiectasis, lung abscess, bronchopneumonia and aspergillosis, carcinoma of lung, surgical lesion extent, use and complications of surgical incisions like anterolateral thoracotomy, posterolateral thoracotomy and median sternotomy, postoperative management of patients with segmentectomy, lobectomy, pneumonectomy, pleuropneumonectomy and tracheostomy, principles of various ventilators and their uses, pre- operative assessment and management of the patient posted for thoracotomy, postoperative procedures like management of endotracheal/endonasal tubes tracheal suction, weaning the patient from the ventilator, extubation technique and postextubation care.

Chapter Six: Describes about management of a patient care after myocardial infarction.

Chapter Seven: Management of a patient with chronic obstructive airway disease includes obstructive lung disease.

Chapter Eight: Cardiac rehabilitation.

Chapter Nine: Pulmonary rehabilitation.

Chapter Ten: Cardiopulmonary resuscitation.

Chapter Eleven: Relaxation techniques.

Chapter Twelve: Breathing control and techniques.

Chapter Thirteen: Posture.

Chapter Fourteen: Total body exercises.

Glossary.

Any suggestions from the teachers and students will be highly appreciated so that further improvement in the information can be made in the subsequent editions in the light of the same.

GB Madhuri
drmadhuri11@gmail.com

Preface to the First Edition

The book titled *Textbook of Physiotherapy for Cardio-respiratory Cardiac Surgery and Thoracic Surgery Conditions* has been design to cater to the needs of the bachelor students of physiotherapy especially in their third and final years. This book is also useful to the professionals of physiotherapy, rehabilitation and other paramedics.

The book has been prepared as per the curriculum and requirement of degree course in India and also abroad. Books on this subject are yet not abundantly available. Very few textbooks are existing in the market which are written by foreign authors.

Physiotherapy is an essential and basic subject for the undergraduate as well as postgraduate courses. The book has been written in a systemic manner and opts a very simple approach in presenting the text. Recently, lots of advances have taken place in cardio-thoracic field. Utmost efforts have been made to cover all the necessary aspects of this subject. All the chapters have been written in a very simple and clearly expressed style.

Physiotherapy is an ever advancing field. The recent advances have made this subject very interesting and it is playing an important role in health care world. I have tried my best to make this book updated starting from introduction to recent advances. To make more informative, Glossary and Bibliography are given at the end of the book.

Any suggestions from the teachers and students will be highly appreciated for the further improvement which can be made in next edition.

GB Madhuri

Acknowledgments

I am indebted to Mr G Ananda Rao, my father for inspiring me and encouraging me at every step of my life.

I am thankful to my beautiful daughters Manasvini Santhoshi and Juhika Santhoshi for always supporting me and motivating for writing this book and endured two years of emotional stress while I was deeply engrossed in preparing this book.

While preparing this book, I have utilized the knowledge of consultants from many books and authors. I wish to express my appreciation and gratitude to all of them who helped me with their valuable suggestions in this venture.

My special thanks to my family who encouraged and supported me and my thoughts to bring out this book perfectly and professionally.

I owe my special thanks to Shri Jitendar P Vij (Group Chairman) of M/s Jaypee Brothers Medical Publishers (P) Ltd, New Delhi, India and whole publishing team for this book in such a nice manner.

Contents

1. **Anatomy** 1
   - Pleurae
   - The Lung
   - Bronchial Tree
   - Bronchopulmonary Segments
   - The Bony Thorax and Lungs
   - The Bony Cage and its Conditions
   - Thorax and its Movements
   - Respiration and its Muscles
   - The Heart and ECG

2. **Physiology** 28
   - The Respiration, Respiratory Centers, and Chemoreceptors
   - Blood Pressure
   - The Cough Reflex
   - Breathing, Lung Compliance, and Airway Resistance
   - The Diffusion, Ventilation, and Perfusion
   - The Energy Expenditure
   - Pulmonary Function Assessment
   - Cardiovascular Stress Testing
   - Arrhythmia and Syncope
   - Syncope and its Management
   - Electrocardiograph

3. **Cardiac Surgery: Closed Heart Conditions and their Physical Therapy Management** 77
   - Acquired Conditions
     - Mitral Stenosis
     - Aortic Stenosis
   - Congenital Conditions
     - Patent Ductus Arteriosus
     - Coarctation of Aorta
   - Physical Therapy Management for Closed Heart conditions

4. **Cardiac Surgery: Open Heart Surgery Conditions and their Physical Therapy Management** 91
   - Congenital Conditions
     - Atrial Septal Defect
     - Ventricular Septal Defect
     - Pulmonary Stenosis
     - Tetralogy of Fallot
     - Transposition of Great Vessels
     - Arteriovenous Malformation

- Acquired Conditions
  - Mitral Stenosis
  - Mitral Regurgitation
  - Aortic Stenosis
  - Aortic Regurgitation
  - Coronary Artery Disease or Ischemic Heart Disease
  - Angina Pectoris
  - Cardiac Failure
- Cardiac Rehabilitation Program for Acquired Open Heart Conditions

5. **Thoracic Surgery** 123
   - Fracture Ribs
   - Flail Chest
   - Stove in Chest
   - Pneumothorax
   - Hemothorax
   - Hemopneumothorax
   - Lung Contusion and Laceration
   - Pulmonary Laceration
   - Injury to Heart, Great Vessels, and Bronchus
   - Empyema
   - Pulmonary Tuberculosis
   - Pott's Disease/Pott's Paraplegia/Pott's Spine/Tuberculosis Spondylitis
   - Tuberculoma
   - Bronchiectasis Sicca
   - Bronchostenosis
   - Massive Hemoptysis
   - Suppurative Lesions of the Lung
   - Carcinoma of Lung
   - Thoracic Surgery
   - Postoperative Complications
   - Incisions, Indications, Contraindications, and Complications
   - Ventilators
   - Preoperative Assessment and Management of a Patient Posted for Thoracotomy
   - Pulmonary Rehabilitation
   - Endotracheal/Endonasal Tubes

6. **Myocardial Infarction—Management and Physical Therapy Intervention** 209

7. **Chronic Obstructive Airway Disease—Management and Physical Therapy Intervention** 218

8. **Cardiac Rehabilitation** 231

Contents

9. Pulmonary Rehabilitation 256
10. Cardiopulmonary Resuscitation 302
11. Relaxation Techniques 308
12. Breathing Control Techniques 312
13. Posture 317
14. Total Body Exercises, Muscles and their Functions 321
    Glossary *330*
    Index *333*

Anatomy

CHAPTER 1

PLEURAE

The pleura is one of the two membranes around the lung. These two membranes are called parietal pleura and visceral pleura. The visceral pleura envelops the lung, whereas parietal pleura lines the inner chest wall. There is pleural fluid in between parietal and visceral pleura. It helps as a lubricant between parietal and visceral pleura. The pleura forms a two-layered membranous pleural sac. There are two pleural sacs on either side of the mediastinum.

The pleural cavity is the thin fluid-filled space between parietal and visceral pleura. The cavity of the thorax contains the right and left pleural cavity that are completely invaginated and occupied by the lungs. The pleural cavities are separated by a thick median partition called the mediastinum. The heart lies in the mediastinum.

Layers of Pleura

- The outer layer is called parietal pleura
- The inner layer is called visceral or pulmonary pleura

Pleural Cavity

The space in between the outer and inner layers of pleura is called pleural cavity.

Nerve Supply

Pleura is supplied by intercostal and phrenic nerves.

Blood Supply

Pleura is supplied by intercostal artery, internal thoracic artery, and musculophrenic artery.

Venous Drainage

Pleura is supplied by azygos vein and internal thoracic vein.

Lymphatic Drainage

Bronchopulmonary lymph nodes.

APPLIED ANATOMY

- **Paracentesis thoracis**: Aspiration of any fluid from the pleural cavity is called paracentesis thoracis. It is done at the 6th intercostal space.
- **Pleurisy**: This is inflammation of the pleura.
- **Pleural effusion**: It is the collection of fluid in the pleural cavity.
- **Pneumothorax**: Presence of air in the pleural cavity.
- **Hemothorax**: Presence of blood in the pleural cavity.
- **Hydropneumothorax**: Presence of both fluid and air in the pleural cavity.
- **Empyema**: Presence of pus in the pleural cavity.

THE LUNG

The lungs are the pair of respiratory organs situated in the thoracic cavity. The right and left lungs are separated by the mediastinum. Lungs are spongy in texture and mottled black in color. The right lung weighs about 625 g and the left lung 575 g. The right lung is 50 g heavier than the left lung.

Features

Each lung is conical in shape and has an upper end called apex. The lower end called base. The base rests on the diaphragm. Each lung has three borders and two surfaces. The borders are anterior, posterior, and inferior. The surfaces are: costal and medial. The medial surface, in turn, is divided into vertebral and mediastinum surfaces.

Fissures and Lobes

The lungs are divided into lobes by fissures. The right lung has three lobes and two fissures and left lung has two lobes and one fissure. The right lung is divided into three lobes [superior (upper), middle and inferior (lower)] lobes by two fissures (horizontal and oblique). The left lung is divided into two lobes [superior (upper) and inferior (lower)] by oblique fissure.

BRONCHIAL TREE

The bronchial tree is formed by trachea, bronchi and its branches. The trachea divides at the level of lower border of the fourth thoracic vertebra into two primary or principal bronchi. Each principal bronchus is divided into right and left bronchus. The right bronchus is divided into three secondary bronchi or lobar bronchi for the three lobes of the right lung. Each secondary bronchus is divided into tertiary or segmental bronchi, one for each bronchopulmonary segment. There are ten bronchopulmonary segments in the right lung and eight in the left lung. The tertiary bronchioles, in turn, are divided into terminal bronchiole, which, in turn, is divided into respiratory bronchiole or pulmonary unit. Each pulmonary unit consists of alveolar ducts, atria, air saccules, and pulmonary alveoli.

Functions of Bronchial Tree

Helps in air conduction in to the lungs and gaseous transportation.

Arterial Supply

Bronchial arteries.

Venous Drainage

Bronchial veins.

Lymphatic Drainage

Bronchopulmonary nodes.

Nerve Supply

The bronchial tree is supplied by both sympathetic and parasympathetic nervous system. They are T2-T5 and vagus nerve.

BRONCHOPULMONARY SEGMENTS

The bronchopulmonary segment is a subdivision of lobe of lung. It is a well-defined section of the lung, each of which is aerated by tertiary or segmental bronchus. Each of the segment is pyramidal in shape. The right lung has eight bronchopulmonary segments and left lung has seven bronchopulmonary segments. As the the right lung has three lobes, the following are the bronchopulmonary segments for each lobe. They are
- The upper lobe has apical, anterior, and posterior bronchopulmonary segments.
- The middle lobe has medial and lateral bronchopulmonary segments.
- The lower lobe has superior basal, anterior basal, posterior basal, and lateral basal bronchopulmonary segments.

The left lung has two lobes. The upper lobe has two subdivisions. They are superior division and lingular division. Both has two bronchopulmonary segments. The following are the bronchopulmonary segments:

- The upper lobe: superior division—the bronchopulmonary segments are apicoposterior and anterior. The lingular division bronchopulmonary segments are superior and inferior.
- The lower lobe has three bronchopulmonary segments. They are superior, anteromedial basal and lateral basal.

Clinical Significance

1. The infection to the individual segment will remain restricted to it
2. Bronchogenic carcinoma and tuberculosis spread from one segment to the other
3. Surgical removal of the segment is called segmental resection. In case of lung abscess or bronchiectasis, the infection is drained by postural drainage
4. Visualizing the interior of the bronchi through an instrument passed through the mouth and trachea. The instrument is called bronchoscope, and the procedure is called bronchoscopy.

THE BONY THORAX AND LUNGS

The bony thorax is the skeletal part of the chest. It is made up of sternum, 12 pairs of ribs and 12 thoracic vertebra. It has vital organs like lungs, heart.

Functions

1. Protects lungs and heart
2. Support pleural cavity and diaphragm during respiration

Thorax: The thorax consist of chest and upper portion of the trunk. The thorax is supported by a skeletal framework called thoracic cage.

Thoracic cage: It is cage like structure that surrounds chest organs like lungs and heart and upper abdomen. The lungs are principle organ of respiration and heart is the principal organ of circulation.

Chest: The chest has thoracic cavity. It has three parts. They are two pleural cavities containing lungs and the space between the pleural cavities is called mediastinum. The mediastinum has heart, trachea, esophagus, thymus and lymph nodes.

Trunk cavities: There are two major cavities. They are thoracic cavity and abdominal pelvic cavity. These two cavities separated by the diaphragm. The diaphragm is a muscle that contracts and relaxes with respiration. The diaphragm is divides the thorax into an upper part called the thorax and a lower part called the abdomen.

Thoracic Cage

Formation

The thoracic cage is an osseocartilaginous elastic cage. The thoracic cage is formed anteriorly by the sternum and posteriorly by the 12th thoracic vertebrae and the intervertebral disk and on either side by 12 ribs with their cartilages. Each rib articulates posteriorly with the vertebral column.

Functions

The thoracic cage is designed primarily for increasing and decreasing the intrathoracic pressure so that air is sucked into the lung during inspiration and expelled during expiration.

Ribs

Ribs are the long curved bones form thoracic cage. There are 12 pairs of ribs.

Function

Respiration.

Types

Three types:
a. *True ribs:* 1 to 7 are called true ribs because the true ribs articulate anteriorly with the sternum through their cartilages called true or vertebra sternal ribs.
b. *False ribs:* 8, 9, 10 are false ribs because the false ribs articulate by joining the next higher costal cartilages called vertebrochondral ribs. These ribs form the costal margin.
c. *Floating ribs:* 11, 12 are called floating or vertebral ribs because ribs are free anteriorly.

Shape of the Thorax

The thorax resembles a truncated cone—narrow above and broad below. The narrow upper end is continuous with the root of the neck from which it is partly separated by the suprapleural membrane called Sibson's fascia. The broad lower end is separated from the abdomen by the diaphragm that is concave downward. The upper part of the thoracic cavity appears broad due to shoulders, and the lower part has an abdominal cavity separated by diaphragm that is a dome-shaped structure with concavity downward.

The transverse section of the thorax in adults is kidney shaped and normally oval in shape. The ribs are oblique, and their movement alternately increases and decreases the diameter of the thorax.

Respiration

There are two types of respiration:
1. Abdominal
2. Thoracic

The inspiration and expiration that occur due to the expansion of the chest are called thoracic respiration. Apart from this, there is also abdominal respiration. In females, respiration is thoracoabdominal, and in males, it is abdominothoracic respiration, in infants and toddlers, the thorax is circular, and the ribs are horizontal so the respiration occurs by diaphragm so it is purely abdominal.

APPLIED ANATOMY

The chest wall of a child is highly elastic so fracture of the ribs is rare. In adults because of direct and indirect violence, e.g., crushing, injury causes fractures to the ribs. The rib can be easily fractured at its weakest point located at the angle. The upper two and lower two ribs can escape from injuries because the clavicles protect the upper ones, whereas the floating ribs protect the lower ones.

A cervical rib is an extra rib attached to C7 vertebrae, which is estimated to occur in 0.5% of population. This cervical rib exerts pressure on the lower trunk of the brachial plexus and produces symptoms such as paresthesia along the ulnar border of the forearm and wasting the small muscles of the hand.

The Inlet of the Thorax or Superior Aperture of the Thorax

The narrow upper end of the thorax that is continuous with the neck is called the inlet of the thorax. It is kidney shaped.

Diameters

The anteroposterior diameter is about 2 inch, and transverse diameter is about 4–5 inch.

Boundaries of the Thorax

Anterior border: Upper border of the manubrium sterni
Posterior border: Superior surface of the body of the first thoracic vertebrae
On each side: First rib with the cartilage.

Diaphragm of the Inlet of the Thorax

The diaphragm is in two halves. They are right and left halves with a cleft in between. Each half is known as Sibson's fascia or suprapleural membrane. This is triangular in shape. It partly separates thorax from the neck.

Structures Passing through the Inlet

The viscera passing through the inlet of the thorax are trachea, esophagus, apices of lungs (with pleura), and the remains of the thymus.

Arterial Supply of the Thorax

- **Right side:** Brachiocephalic artery
- **Left side:** Subclavian artery

Venous Supply of the Thorax

- **Right side:** Right brachiocephalic vein
- **Left side:** Left brachiocephalic vein

Nervous Supply of the Thorax

Right and left side: Phrenic nerve, vagus nerve, sympathetic trunk, and first thoracic nerves.

Muscles Supplying the Thorax

Sternohyoid, sternothyroid, and longus colli.

APPLIED ANATOMY

Thoracic Inlet Syndrome
The subclavian artery and the first thoracic nerves arch over the first rib. These structures may be pulled or pressed by the cervical rib or by variation in the insertion of the scalenus anterior so symptoms will be vascular or neural.

Outlet of the Thorax: The Inferior Aperture
It is the broad end of the thorax that surrounds the upper part of the abdominal cavity and is separated by diaphragm.

Boundaries

- **Anteriorly:** Infra-sternal angle between two costal margins
- **Posteriorly:** Inferior surface of the body of the 12th thoracic vertebra
- **On each side:** Costal margin formed by the cartilage of 7th, 8th, 9th, 10th, 11th, and 12th ribs.

Diaphragm Passing through the Outlet

The outlet is closed by a large musculotendinous partition called the diaphragm. The diaphragm is a thoracoabdominal organ structure that separates the thorax from the abdomen.

Structures Passing through the Outlet—Large Openings in the Diaphragm

1. **Vena caval opening:** This is at T8 vertebra level and transmits inferior vena cava, branches of right phrenic nerve.
2. **Esophageal opening:** This is at T10 vertebra level and transmits esophagus, gastric (vagus nerve), gastric artery, and esophageal veins.
3. **Aortic opening:** This is at T12 vertebra level and transmits aorta, thoracic duct, and azygos vein.

▌THE BONY CAGE AND ITS CONDITIONS

The following conditions are discussed with physical therapy management. They are:
a. Cervical rib
b. Rickets
c. Osteomalacia
d. Pigeon chest
e. Funnel chest
f. Scoliosis
g. Kyphosis

Cervical Rib

The cervical rib is a extra rib coming out from the cervical spine location above 1st rib. The extra cervical rib is seen in 0.5% of individuals. The rib exerts pressure on the lower trunk of brachial plexus that arches over the rib and produces paresthesia along the ulnar border of the forearm and wasting of the muscles of the hand supplied by T1 nerve root. Vascular changes may occur. This extra rib is also associated with the spinal anomalies.

Types of Anomalies

These are the main varieties:
1. A complete rib often containing a false joint in its length articulates anteriorly with the manubrium or first rib.
2. A free end of rib expands into a large bony mass.
3. A rib ending in a tapering point.
4. A fibrous band loosely incorporated into scalenus medius muscle. At their exit from the neck, the brachial plexus and subclavian artery pass through a narrow triangle.

By the interposition of a cervical rib, the base of the triangle is raised by the height of one vertebra. The subclavian artery and first dorsal nerve become angulated as they pass over the new floor of cervical vertebra rather than the first thoracic rib.

Pathology of the Vascular Symptoms

The lumen of the subclavian artery becomes constricted. Dilatation of the first 2-4 cm of the artery occurs distal to the constriction. With the poststenotic dilatation, clotting occurs. Position of the thrombus may become detached and give rise to an emboli or embolus. Proximal extension of the thrombus can occur so that vertebral artery may be involved and cerebrovascular emboli episodes occur.

Clinical Types

1. **Cervical rib with local symptoms:** Patient will have a lump in the lower part of the neck that may be visible more commonly because of the tenderness in the supraclavicular fossa. On palpation, lump is found to be hard, bony, and totally fixed.
2. **Cervical rib with vascular symptoms:** Vascular symptoms occur only when cervical rib is complete. Pain is felt in the upper arm and forearm. Pain is caused by the use of arms and relieved by rest. The type of pain is similar to ischemic muscle pain.
   - *Temperature and color change:* Hand on the affected side tends to be colder and turns pale and blue.
   - *Radial pulse:* The pulse is full with the good blood circulation. But if the circulation is interrupted due to many reasons the pulse can be feeble or absent. Distal part of the subclavian artery could be auscultated. In this scenario, patients complain of numbness of fingers, ulceration, and gangrene.
3. **Cervical rib with nerve pressure symptoms:** The symptoms can range from cervical spondylosis, carpal tunnel syndrome and scalene syndrome with symptoms like pain, tingling sensation in forearm and arm and wasting of muscles like thenar muscles and hypothenar muscles of hand secondary to angulation of the first dorsal nerve.

Treatment

Treatment includes extraperitoneal excision of cervical rib and bony prominence of the first rib and sympathetic denervation of the upper limb.

Differential Diagnosis

1. In the region of intervertebral foramen there is pressure on the cervical roots caused by lateral protrusion of the intervertebral disks
2. *Carpal tunnel syndrome:* It is the condition seen with the compression of lateral and medial cord of brachial plexus causing symptoms like numbness, paresthesia or wasting of thenar eminence which includes thenar muscles like flexor pollicis brevis, abductor pollicis brevis, opponens pollicis brevis and adductor pollicis.
3. Hypothenar wasting arising from angulation of ulnar nerve behind the elbow or compression of the medial cord of the brachial plexus causing paresthesia or wasting of hypothenar eminence or muscles like flexor digiti minimi, abdcutor digiti minimi, opponens digiti minimi and palmaris brevis.
4. *Motor neuron disease:* It affects motor neurons of brain and spinal cord causing weakness, wasting and fasciculation. It is a life-threatening disorder.
   Types: There are four types of motor neuron disease:
   a. Primary lateral sclerosis
   b. Progressive bulbar palsy
   c. Amyotrophic lateral sclerosis
   d. Progressive muscle atrophy
5. *Syringomyelia:* It is a chronic condition with fluid-filled cavities in the spinal cord causing compression and damage of the spinal cord.

On Examination

a. Pain in the neck
b. Decreased range of motion in the neck
c. Weakness in the upper extremity
d. Pins and needle sensation in the upper extremity

Treatment

The treatment can be divided as: i) conservative treatment and ii) surgical treatment.

Physical therapy management:

S. No.	Aims of PT	Plan of PT
1.	To reduce pain	Thermotherapy
2.	To educated the patient	Postural education

Contd...

Contd...

S. No.	Aims of PT	Plan of PT
3.	To improve muscle strength	Strengthening exercises to all muscles of neck, shoulder girdle and upper limb
4.	To reduce neck and shoulder girdle stiffness	Soft tissue massage for trapezius muscles and stretching
5.	To reduce nerve impingement	Soft tissue mobilization Grade 1 and 2 for reducing pain Grade 3 and 4 for improving range of motion

Surgical treatment: If the physical therapy treatment does not bring relief of the symptoms then surgical treatment is indicated where the cervical rib or first rib are removed by cutting the anterior or middle scalene muscles.

Rickets or Rachitic Rosary/Osteomalacia

Definition

This is a metabolic disorder. It is seen in children called as rickets and in adults called osteomalacia.

Mechanism

The bone metabolism is impaired due to inadequate absorption of vitamin D, calcium, phosphate causing inadequate bone mineralization.

Rickets

There are three types of rickets:
1. Nutritional
2. Celiac
3. Renal nutritional rickets

Rickets is more common in children below 4 years and occurs due to the deficiency of vitamin D.

Pathology
1. Defective absorption of calcium from the gut.
2. Lowering of calcium and phosphate in tissue fluid.
3. Broadening of metaphysis and widening of epiphysis in the long axis of bone.
4. There is a poor deposition of calcium in zone of calcification and poor mineralization of spongy bone.

5. Bone becomes soft and pliable and deforms easily on weight bearing and on stress.

Clinical Features
1. Child will be irritable
2. Child sweats excessively
3. Child growth gets stunned
4. Fontanelle remains unclosed after 2 years
5. There will be bossing over frontal and parietal bone called cross burn appearance
6. The chest shows pigeon chest deformity
7. Beading at costochondral junction occurs called rachitic rosary

Treatment
Medical management: Vitamin D and Ca supplements and proper sun exposure.

Physical therapy management: Patient and family education—Vitamin D, calcium supplements and proper sun exposure.

Osteomalacia

Definition: The osteomalacia is seen in the adults. It is the condition with impairment of bone metabolism due to inadequate absorption of vitamin D, calcium and phosphate causing inadequate bone mineralization.

Clinical Features:
1. Fatigue
2. Proximal muscle pain/bone pain
3. Hip pain
4. Muscle weakness
5. Waddling gait
6. First sign is fracture then bone deformity
7. Difficulty with sit to stand, carrying load, climbing stairs and activities of daily living

Medical management: Vitamin D, calcium and phosphate supplements, proper sun exposure.

Physical therapy management: The main focus of exercise is extension bias. That means the patient is comfortable doing extension exercises and flexion exercises should be avoided like flexion and twisting because they can lead to spinal compression fractures.

S. No.	Aims of physical therapy	Plan of physical therapy
1.	To increase muscle strengthen	Exercises for whole body using weights, bands
2.	To increase postural awareness to improve balance and decrease falls	Postural exercises like weight-bearing exercises like ambulation
3.	To teach activities of daily living	Sit to stand, carrying loads, climbing stairs, etc.
4.	To teach extension exercises	Chin tucks, scapular retraction, thoracic exercises, hip extension, etc.
5.	To prevent fractures	Avoid high impact exercises, lifting heavy weights
6.	To educate the patient	Healthy diet, well fitted shoes, good lighting on the stairs, regular eye check up
7.	To prevent falls	Static and dynamic balance exercises and activities

Pigeon Chest or Pigeon Breast or Pectus Carinatum

Definition

It is the forward projection of the sternum like a keel of a boat and flattening of chest wall on either side.

It is an outgrowth of sternum. It is also called protrusion deformity of the chest characterized by protrusion of the sternum that causes upward curve in the lower costal cartilage at the level of 4–8 Ribs.

Causes

1. Severe asthma in the childhood
2. Rickets
3. Sometimes no cause
4. Malformation in mobility of intrauterine life and sternum comes anteriorly because of the movement of the ribs.

Symptoms

1. Exertional dyspnea
2. Cardiac arrhythmias
3. The reduced flexibility of the chest wall limits chest expansion during inspiration by the anterior displaced sternum and abnormal cartilages.

Deformity

It is of three types:
1. Most common is anterior displacement of the body of the sternum with symmetrical concavity of the costal cartilage.
2. Asymmetrical deformities consist of unilateral displacement of the costal cartilage.
3. The least common is chondromanubrial deformity.

Treatment

Surgical treatment: The inferior mammary or horizontal or transverse incision is made through the route of suprasternal notch and infrasternal notch and separates sternum. The chondral pieces are taken out and pinned them into a straight piece. Cartilage grows rapidly in 3 months. It brings the sternum down.

Funnel Chest

It is the most common congenital deformity of the sternum. It is an excessive, misdirected growth of the lower costal cartilages. Funnel chest is a congenital condition. The rapid growth of the sternum is seen in this condition and the severity of disease can increase with time causing sternal depression.

Causes

1. Congenital
2. Malformation or misdirection of growth of ribs during intrauterine period.

Clinical Features

1. The body and the lower end of the sternum are curved back
2. The heart is displaced to the left and compressed between the sternum and the vertebral column
3. There will be a disturbance of the cardiac function
4. The deformity may resist chest expansion and reduce vital capacity
5. Recurrent lower respiratory tract infection and asthma may be seen in patients with this deformity
6. Scoliosis is associated with anterior chest wall deformity
7. Paraspinal muscle imbalances are present
8. Asymmetry causes pneumatic thoracic pressure
9. The thoracic curve is involved between T4 and T9

10. Mitral valve prolapse is seen
11. Cardiac and respiratory functions are reduced
12. Excessive angulation is seen
13. The restful environment can decrease the severity of the funnel chest deformity in children
14. The severity of the problem increases physical activity
15. This limits social life.

Treatment

Surgical treatment: Horizontal incision is made, sternum is separated, and the chondral pieces are taken out. They are pinned by keeping sternum straight, followed by suturing and then closing perichondrium, muscles, and skin. The cartilage grows rapidly in 3 months.

Spinal Curve

The spine consists of two curves:
1. **Primary curve**: At birth, only primary curves are present. This is concave anteriorly and convex posteriorly and present in the thoracic and sacral region.
2. **Secondary curve**: In the adult, this along with the primary curve is present. This is concave posteriorly and convex anteriorly and present in the cervical and lumbar region.

Functions of spinal curves
1. These curves increase the strength of the spine.
2. They help to maintain balance in the upright position.
3. These help in shock absorption.
4. These help in protecting the spinal cord from injury.

APPLIED ANATOMY

- **Abnormal curves**: These can occur due to congenital problems or due to postural differences.
- **Scoliosis**: This is the lateral bending of the vertebral column that usually affects the thoracic region.
- **Kyphosis**: The thoracic curve gets exaggerated due to rounded shoulders.
- **Lordosis**: This is an exaggeration of the lumbar curve.

Scoliosis

A lateral curvature of the spine that exceeds by 10° from the normal is termed scoliosis.

Types

It is basically of two types:
1. Postural or nonstructural scoliosis
2. Structural scoliosis

1. **Postural or nonstructural scoliosis:** This is grade-I scoliosis. This occurs without any bony changes or muscular weakness.
Causes:
- Impairment of the reflex mechanism.
- Wrong postural habits, e.g., standing with stress on one leg or psychological factors. The postural scoliosis may get organized into a structural one, due to secondary soft tissue contractures in muscles and ligaments on the concave side of the curve.

2. **Structural scoliosis:** This comes under grades II and III. In this type, there is a defect in the bone that results in contractures of the soft tissue on the concave side of the curve and reciprocal stretching on the concave side.
Classification:
a. Postural or idiopathic scoliosis
b. Paralytic scoliosis
c. Congenital scoliosis

a. **Postural or idiopathic scoliosis:** This is divided into four types:
  i. *Infantile:* The onset of this is at the age of 3 years. Usually, there is a spontaneous resolution of the curve. If the curve progresses, then there is a need for an early surgical intervention.
  ii. *Juvenile:* The age of onset is between 3 and 10 years. Rapid progression of the curve occurs due to the growing age. If bracing fails to control the deterioration, surgery becomes necessary.
  iii. *Adolescent:* The age of onset is between 10 and 20 years. If this is detected earlier, acceptable correction is achieved by bracing.
  iv. *Adult:* The age of onset is over 20 years. Scoliosis may develop as a result of disk degeneration. When the deterioration is rapidly progressive, surgery may be indicated.
b. **Paralytic scoliosis:** This occurs in conditions such as poliomyelitis, cerebral palsy, or spina bifida. This is complicated by the greater degree of muscle imbalance and growing age complications. Scoliosis will rapidly deteriorate in these children. Surgery becomes necessary where there is a rapid progression of the curve.

c. **Congenital scoliosis:** This scoliosis occurs by birth. It is of milder and severe forms. The milder form is treated with a brace, whereas the severe form needs a surgery.

The Course and Prognosis

The course depends on the age of onset, time of detection, site of the primary curve, and the treatment given. If the onset is at an early age, the curve tends to increase with age till the end of the skeletal growth. The prognosis will be poor if affects thoracic curve because it interferes the breathing efficiency. The thoracolumbar or lumbar curves will compensate well.

Prevention

Prevention plays a very important role:
1. Early detection plays an important role in the prevention of scoliosis.
2. Screening program of all the children between the age group of 10 and 14 years is necessary because they are more vulnerable.
3. Parents can also play an important role in the early detection of a scoliotic curve. So education of the parents on observational techniques may be helpful.

Treatment

Curve <40°: Conservative treatment is sufficient in growing children. The treatment can be given in the following ways:
1. **Active correction:** This is a postural correction, which is again divided into grades I, II, and III.
    a. *Grade I—Management of postural scoliosis:* The correction of the deformity is obtained by a progressive reduction of the bad posture.
        - General body relaxation
        - Posture maintenance
        - Free mobility exercises to the whole spine, spinal extensor exercises, and abdominal exercises
        - Deep breathing exercises
        - Balance exercise
        - Stretching of the soft tissues
        - After the correction, the patient should be advised to continue with exercises avoiding especially the positions and the activities prone to produce the existing deformity
        - The patient must report regularly for screening.

b. *Grade II:* The curves are associated with the compensatory curves so need a brace called Milwaukee or Boston brace to prevent deterioration of the curve and to maintain correction with active exercise. This brace immobilizes the spine and maintains a stretching effect.

   Exercise program:
   - Mobility exercises are important as the spine remains immobilized in brace.
   - Deep breathing exercises are also important as the expansion of the ribs is limited due to the brace.
   - Lumbar lordosis is associated with these curves so correction of the anterior pelvic tilt is important.
   - Correction of the major curve is also achieved by putting a pad over a rib hump on the convex side of the curve in the brace.
   - Repeated stretching exercises for the hip flexors and hamstrings are important as these have a tendency to shorten due to the pelvic tilt.
   - Hanging in head suspension apparatus or on the stall bars can provide effective stretch to the whole spine.
   - The whole program and the brace need to be continued for longtime. As the child grows, brace needs repeated adjustment and needs to be continued till the child attains skeletal maturity. It can be taken gradually thereafter. The brace needs to be worn day and night except during the exercise program of spinal mobilization and deep breathing exercise. The thoracic flexion exercise should be taught with the brace on position because this reduces vertebral rotation.

   c. *Grade III—Severe structural curves:* These curves are greater than 40° and need a surgical intervention.

2. **Passive correction:** Hanging is the best method, e.g., suspension apparatus. Two physiotherapists give axial traction. One will be grasping the pelvis and gives traction toward the legs, while the other grasps the chin and gives traction toward the occiput.
3. **Maintenance of correction:** The most important aspect is to educate the patient to maintain the correction by active efforts or with the help of spinal brace. The patient needs education for continuous awareness of an exact methodology.

Kyphosis

Kyphosis or kyphosis arcuata or round back is the exaggeration of the posterior spinal curve and is generally localized to the dorsal

spine or thoracic spine. The back will be rounded, the head is carried forward, and the chest is flattened. This results in typical round shoulders with excessive protrusion of the scapula.
1. **School age:** The habitual posture at the school is the main cause. Mental and physical fatigue could also precipitate such habitual postural tendencies. It could also be developed as a result of undetected defects of vision or hearting.
2. **Adolescent age:** This occurs as a result of arthritis, rheumatism, lung affections, e.g., emphysema, vertebral disease, and habitual bad posture.
3. **Old age:** This occurs as a result of previous bad posture, muscular weakness, degeneration, and disease of the vertebral bodies and disks.

Deformity

The scoliosis deformity is divided in to three categories. They are:
1. **First-degree kyphosis:** Progress of the deformity is from first to third degree. A habitual posture is the precipitating factor. There is no imbalance in the muscle; if this is not corrected at this stage, it progresses to the second stage.

The changes are as follows:
- The pectoral muscles become short, thereby restricting the chest expansion resulting in the reduced respiratory function.
- The longitudinal back muscles, rhomboids, and the middle trapezius are unduly stretched and weakened with the loss of tone.
- The posterior ligaments are lengthened, and the anterior structures are shortened. This causes an increase in posterior laxity and a typical kyphotic deformity.
- The wedging of the vertebral bodies may occur in the adolescent stage of the growth period. This gets organized into the third-degree deformity, which is a difficult syndrome.

Kyphosis can also occur due to the tuberculosis, ankylosing spondylitis, Scheuermann's disease, or congenital anomalies.

Physiotherapy Management

1. **First-degree kyphosis:**
   a. Relaxation
   b. Stretching exercises
   c. Posture maintenance
2. **Second- and third-degree kyphosis:** The wrong adaptations of the soft tissues are in the advanced stage. Milwaukee brace is prescribed with pads applied on the posterior upright.

Exercises

The exercises are done with the brace on, and the patient should be encouraged to put the maximum pressure over these posterior pads. This stretches the shoulder, shoulder girdle, and kyphotic curve. Sustenance of the active stretching is very important.

It is difficult to achieve enough correction, but it certainly helps in preventing further deterioration of the curve. Exercise to improve the mobility and respiration reduces the overall impact of the deformity.

Surgical and Postsurgical Management

After the surgical correction is done, it involves gradual controlled halo-traction for several weeks. Bone grafting may be necessary to maintain the correction achieved through traction. Spinal stabilization is required through anterior approach in cases with severe kyphotic curves, tuberculous lesions, and spinal cord decompression.

THORAX AND ITS MOVEMENTS

Respiratory Movements

The lungs expand passively during inspiration and retract during expiration. These movements are governed by the following two factors:

1. Alteration in the capacity of the thorax is brought about by movements of the thoracic wall. Increase in volume of the thoracic cavity creates negative intrathoracic pressure that sucks air into the lungs. Movements of the thoracic wall occur chiefly at the costovertebral and manubriosternal joints.
2. Elastic recoil of the pulmonary alveoli and of the thoracic wall expels air from the lungs during expiration.

Principles of Movement

1. Each rib may be regarded as a lever, the fulcrum of which lies just lateral to the tubercle. Because of the disproportion in the length of the two arms of the lever, the slight movements at the vertebral end of the ribs are significantly magnified at the anterior end.
2. The anterior end of the rib is lower than the posterior end. Therefore during the elevation of the rib, the anterior end also moves forward. This occurs in the vertebrosternal ribs. So anterior–posterior of the thorax is increased. There are up and down movements. The second to sixth ribs along with this body

of the sternum also move up and down, which is called pump-handle movements.
3. The thorax resembles a cone. Consequently, each rib is longer than the next higher rib. On elevation, the larger lower rib comes to occupy the position of the smaller upper rib. This also increases the transverse diameter of the thorax. This is mainly by the bucket handle movements of the vertebrochondral (7th–10th) ribs, partly by elevation of the vertebrosternal ribs. The vertical diameter is increased by the descent of the diaphragm.

Inspiration

The drawing of air into the lungs is called inspiration. There are three types of inspiration:
1. **Quiet inspiration:** In this type of inspiration, the anterior-posterior diameter of the thorax is increased by elevation of the 2nd–6th ribs. The first rib remains fixed. The transverse diameter is increased by elevation of 7th–10th ribs. The vertical diameter is increased by descent of the diaphragm.
2. **Deep inspiration**: In this type of inspiration, the movements during quiet inspiration are increased. The first rib is elevated by scalene and sternocleidomastoid muscles. The concavity of the thoracic spine is reduced by the erector spinae.
3. **Forced inspiration:** In this type of inspiration, all the movements are exaggerated. The scapulae are elevated and fixed by the trapezius, levator scapulae, and the rhomboids muscle so that the serratus anterior and the pectoralis minor muscles may act on the ribs. The action of the erector spinae is increased.

Expiration

The breathing out of air from lungs is called expiration. This is of three types:
1. **Quiet expiration:** This expiration occurs by elastic recoil of the chest wall and pulmonary alveoli. They both help to partly expel the air with the help of abdominal muscle tone.
2. **Deep expiration:** The deep expiration is also called forced expiration is required when normal expiration is not sufficient to expire the complete air so requires the help of expiratory muscles like internal intercostal, external oblique, internal oblique, rectus abdominis and transverse abdominis. The abdominal muscles acts as accessory muscles forces abdominal organs upward against the diaphragm so expiration is possible.

> **APPLIED ANATOMY**
>
> **Dyspnea:** This is also called breathlessness or difficulty in breathing. Such patients will be more comfortable in sitting up, leaning forward, and fixing the arm because the position of the diaphragm is lowest allowing the maximum ventilation, whereas the height of the diaphragm is high on lying down and standing and lowest on sitting down.

RESPIRATION AND ITS MUSCLES

Breathing

The alternate inspiration and expiration of air into and out of the lungs are called breathing.

The muscles that help for breathing are of two types:

1. **Inspiratory muscles:** This muscles contract to draw air into the lungs. The diaphragm plays the most important function, and external intercostal muscles assist with normal quiet breathing. The accessory muscles of respiration are sternocleidomastoid, scalene, pectoralis, and serratus anterior.
2. **Expiratory muscles:** This is a passive process as lung's recoil inward and collapse. Lungs deflate without the effort of muscles. The muscles helping for expiration are internal intercostal, rectus abdominis, external oblique, internal oblique, and transverse abdominis.

Types of Breathing

There are three types of breathing:

1. **Quiet breathing or eupnea:** This type of respiration occurs during rest, and the muscles helping for this are as follows:
   - *Quiet inspiration:* The muscles working are diaphragm and intercostal muscles.
   - *Quiet expiration:* This is a passive process in which inspiratory muscles relax and lungs (pulmonary alveoli) and thoracic wall recoil inward.
2. **Deep breathing:** This type of breathing occurs during exercise or relaxation techniques called diaphragmatic breathing. The muscles helping for inspiration and expiration are as follows:
   - *Inspiration:* Scalene and sternocleidomastoid muscles
   - *Expiration:* Abdominals and latissimus dorsi muscles

   Benefits of deep breathing
   - It reduces stress, tension, and anxiety

- It improves posture
- It gives calming effect
3. **Force breathing or hyperpnea:** This exercise occurs during exercise or singing
   - *Inspiration:* Diaphragm, intercostal, sternomastoid, scalene, serratus anterior, pectoralis minor, erector spinae, alaeque nasi muscles
   - *Expiration:* Abdominals, internal intercostal muscles, and latissimus dorsi muscles, e.g., blowing out candle

APPLIED ANATOMY

1. **Overloading of breathing muscles and respiratory muscle fatigue:** These symptoms are seen in lung disease conditions.
2. **In COPD, cervical SCI and high thoracic SCI:** Increased diaphragmatic breathing is seen with increased use of accessory muscles of respiration.
3. **Diaphragmatic fatigue:** This causes rapid and shallow breathing called paradoxical respiration with increasing rib cage and abdominal movements and decreasing the diaphragmatic muscle contractions.

Treatment

Respiratory muscle training (RMT) increases the entrance and strength of inspiratory and expiratory muscles by breathing against resistance. Resistance training is of two types:
1. **Flow resistance:** Breathing by small opening that increases flow resistance.
2. **Pressure resistance (PR):** Breathing by spring tight/compressed spring located valve that increases PR.

   In both RMTs, resistance can be adjusted according to work out.

   Endurance training or voluntary isocapnic hyperpnea: This includes breathing above normal tidal volume and respiratory rate for 30 minutes.

   Devices for strengthening: Inspiratory muscle training (IMT), expiratory muscle training (EMT), and both IMT and EMT (concurrent).

Types

Power lung: This device trains for PR, IMT, and EMT.
Power breathe: This device trains for PR and IMT.
Ultrabreathe: IMT, FR.
Uses: All these devices help to increase strength, increase diaphragm thickness, and increase fatigue resistance.
Benefits: These devices can be used for patients with multiple diagnoses and athletics.

THE HEART AND ECG

The heart is a conical, hollow muscular organ situated in the middle mediastinum. It is enclosed within the pericardium. It pumps the blood to various parts of the body to meet their nutritive requirement.

The heart is placed obliquely behind the body of the sternum. The heart measures 12 cm in length, 8.5 cm in width and 6 cm in thickness and weighs about 300 g in males and 250 g in females.

External Features

The human heart has four chambers. These are the right and left atria and right and left ventricles. The atria lie above and behind the ventricles. Atria are separated from the ventricles by atrioventricular (AV) groove. The atria are separated from each other by an interatrial groove, whereas the ventricles are separated from each other by an intraventricular groove, which is subdivided into anterior and posterior parts.

Description

The heart has:
Apex: This is directed downward. It is formed by the left ventricle. It is situated in the left fifth intercostal space.
Base: This forms posterior surface and directed backward. It is formed by the left atrium and right atrium.
Surfaces: There are two surfaces:
1. *Anterior or sternocostal surface:* This is formed by the right atrium and right ventricle.
2. *Inferior or diaphragmatic surface:* This is formed by the left ventricle and left atrium.

Borders: The borders of the heart are upper, inferior, right, and left.
Grooves or sulci: The atria are separated from the ventricles by a circular AV or coronary sulcus.

Valves of the Heart

The valves of the heart maintain unidirectional flow of the blood and prevent its regurgitation in the opposite direction. There are two pairs of valves in the heart, one pair of AV valves and another pair of semilunar valves. The right AV valve is known as tricuspid valve because it has three cusps. The left AV valve is known as bicuspid valve because it has two cusps. It is also called mitral valve. The semilunar valve includes the aortic and pulmonary valve, each having three semilunar cusps. The cusps are folds of endocardium, strengthened by an intervening layer of the fibrous tissue. The first heart sound is produced by the closure of the AV valve; the second heart sound is produced by the closure of the semilunar valve.

APPLIED ANATOMY

- The narrowing of the valve orifice due to the fusion of the valve cusps is known as stenosis, e.g., mitral stenosis and aortic stenosis.
- Dilatation of the valve orifice or stiffening of the cusps causes imperfect closure of the valve leading to back flow of the blood. This is known as incompetence or regurgitation, e.g., mitral incompetence or regurgitation and aortic incompetence or regurgitation.

Arterial Supply

The arterial supply is by the right and left coronary artery.

APPLIED ANATOMY

- Myocardial infarction and ventricular fibrillation are the thrombosis of a coronary artery that is a common cause of sudden death in persons in their middle age.
- Angina pectoris is the incomplete obstruction of the coronary artery associated with agonizing pain in the precordial region and goes down on the medial side of the left arm and forearm.

Venous Supply

The venous supply of the heart is by great cardiac veins, middle cardiac veins, small cardiac veins, posterior vein of the left ventricle, oblique vein of left atrium, and right marginal vein. All these drain into the coronary sinus which, in turns, opens into the right atrium. There are two other veins that carry blood directly into right atrium. They are anterior cardiac vein and venae cordis minimae.

Lymphatic Drainage

The two trunks: (1) right trunk ends in the brachiocephalic nodes, and (2) left trunk ends in the tracheobronchial lymph nodes from the lymphatic of the heart.

Nerve Supply of the Heart

Parasympathetic Nerve Supply

This is by vagus nerve. The action is cardioinhibitory. This slows down the stimulation after stimulating.

Sympathetic Nerve Supply

This is by upper 3-5 thoracic segments of the spinal cord. The action is cardioacceleratory. This increases the heart rate after stimulating.

Both sympathetic and parasympathetic nerves form the superficial and deep cardiac plexus. The superficial cardiac plexus is situated below the arch of the aorta, and deep cardiac plexus is situated behind the arch of the aorta.

Clinical Aspects

1. The area of the chest wall overlying the heart is called precordium
2. Tachycardia is an increase in the heart rate
3. Bradycardia is a decrease in the heart rate
4. Arrhythmia is an irregular heart rate
5. Palpitation is a consciousness of the heartbeat.

APPLIED ANATOMY

- Inflammation of the heart can involve more than one layer of the heart
- Inflammation of the pericardium is called pericarditis
- Inflammation of the myocardium is called myocarditis
- Inflammation of the epicardium is called epicarditis
- Right-side heart failure is called congestive cardiac failure
- Right-side heart failure due to lung disease is called cor pulmonale
- The apex beat is on the left side normally; if felt on the right side, it is called dextrocardia
- The incomplete obstruction of the coronary artery causes cardiac pain

Electrical Activity of the Myocardium

Conducting System of the Heart

It is made up of myocardium that is specialized for initiation and conduction of the cardiac impulse.

1. **Sinoatrial node (SA node):** It is also known as a pacemaker of the heart. It generates an impulse at the rate of about 70/min and initiates heart rate. It passes to AV node.
2. **AV node:** This generates an impulse of 60/min.
3. **AV bundle (or bundle of His):** It is only a muscular connection between atrial and ventricular musculature. It is divided into right and left branches. The right branch passes own the right side of the interventricular septum and divides into Purkinje fibers. The left branch descends on the left side of the interventricular septum and divides into Purkinje fibers and is distributed to the left ventricle. The Purkinje fibers form a subendocardial plexus.

APPLIED ANATOMY

- Arrhythmias are the vascular lesion of the heart.
- Cardiac arrhythmia is the defect or damage in the system and in the normal rhythm of contraction.

Electrocardiogram: The record or the registration of electrical activity of cardiac muscle fibers of the heart is called electrocardiogram.

Electrocardiography: This is the technique by which the electrical activities of the heart is studied.

Electrocardiograph: This is the instrument by which the electrical activities of the heart is recorded.

Physiology 2

THE RESPIRATION, RESPIRATORY CENTERS, AND CHEMORECEPTORS

Respiration

Definition

Respiration is a process of breathing. Inhale of oxygen and exhale of carbon dioxide occurs in respiration. Respiration is a chemical process happening in the cells and breathing is the biological process happening between cell and environment through inhaling and exhaling the gases.

Respiratory system has five organs of breathing or five parts of respiration. They are nose/mouth, pharynx, larynx, trachea, bronchi, lungs and diaphragm.

Functions

- Helps in gaseous exchange
- Maintains acid-base balance
- Helps for phonation
- Maintains metabolism.

Control of Respiration

The respiratory center (RC) controls the breathing. RC is located in medulla oblongata. It is the primary control center. The second group is located in pons. Both together functions to control the respiration.

The Respiratory Center

The RC is formed by a group of nerve cells that controls the rate and depth of respiration. The RC receives chemical, neural, and hormonal signals.

Function of Respiratory Center

- Regulates the depth and rate of respiratory movement.
- Maintain rhythm of respiration
- Maintain homeostasis response

Location: RCs are situated in the brainstem in medulla oblongata and pons.

Types: There are 3 major groups of neurons, two are located in medulla, they are dorsal respiratory group is called inspiratory center and ventral respiratory group is called expiratory center and in pons one group called pontine respiratory group which has two areas called pneumatic center which controls the rate and pattern of breathing and apneutic center acts as both stimulation to inspiratory center causing inspiration and inhibitory impulse to expiratory center.

Stimulation: When oxygen, carbon dioxide and pH levels are altered or hormonal changes occurs secondary to stress and anxiety levels then respiratory center is activated and homeostasis is maintained.

Causes: Traumatic brain injury, tumors, drugs like sedatives and opioids cause depression of the respiratory center.

Applied anatomy: Injury to the respiratory center causes respiratory failure.

Treatment: Mechanical ventilation

Prognosis: Poor

Receptors: Breathing is controlled by chemoreceptors. The respiratory receptors are called chemoreceptors. There are two types of chemoreceptors. They are central and peripheral or arterial chemoreceptors.

Chemoreceptors

These are receptors that respond to the changes in the partial pressure of oxygen and carbon dioxide in the blood and cerebrospinal fluid. These are located centrally and peripherally.

Central Chemoreceptors

These receptors are located on the surface of the medulla oblongata and bathed in the cerebrospinal fluid. Aortic and carotid bodies are present in central chemoreceptors, which monitor oxygen concentration in arterial blood, arterial carbon dioxide, and pH. When the arterial partial pressure of carbon dioxide rises even slightly, the central chemoreceptors respond by stimulating the RC. When the ventilation of the lungs increases, the arterial partial pressure of carbon dioxide reduces. The sensitivity of the central chemoreceptors to the raised arterial partial pressure carbon dioxide is the most important factor in maintaining the homeostasis of the blood gases. A small reduction in partial pressure of oxygen has the same effect but less pronounced, but a sustained reduction has a depressed effect.

Peripheral Chemoreceptors

These receptors are situated in the arch of aorta and carotid bodies. The aortic body receptors respond to changes in blood oxygen and carbon dioxide only and carotid body receptors respond to changes in blood oxygen, carbon dioxide and pH levels. These are more sensitive to a small rise in the arterial partial pressure of carbon dioxide and partial pressure of oxygen level. The nerve impulses generated in the peripheral chemoreceptors are conveyed to the medulla and the RC. The stimulation of the chemoreceptors causes increase in the rate and the depth of the breathing, pH levels are decreased, blood circulation is increased, increased ventilation and increased carbon dioxide excretion are seen. These maintain homeostasis and respond to hypoxia (low oxygen), hypercapnia (high carbon dioxide), and hypoglycemia (low glucose).

BLOOD PRESSURE

Definition

It is the force or pressure that the blood exerts on the walls of the blood vessels.

It is the pressure in large arteries of systemic circulation. The normal blood pressure is 120 mm/80 mm Hg. It is systolic/diastolic blood pressure. Systolic BP is the maximum pressure during one heartbeat and diastolic BP is the minimum pressure between two heartbeats. The vital signs of the body are BP, body temperature, oxygen saturation and heart rate (HR). So BP is one of the most important vital signs.

Peripheral resistance: The peripheral resistance is blood pressure divided by cardiac output: PR = BP mm Hg × Cardiac output ML/min.

The pressure in the large arteries varies as the heart contracts and relaxes. BP varies from person to person. The variables influencing BP are age and gender. Blood pressure is regulated by baroreceptors.

Factors Affecting Blood Pressure

The factors, which work together to maintain the BP in normal limits, are as follows:
1. Amount of blood circulating in the blood vessel
2. Cardiac output
3. Elasticity of the large arteries
4. Caliber of the small arterioles called peripheral resistance
5. Arterial stiffness

1. **Amount of blood circulating in the blood vessel:** The amount of the blood in the circulation will be less in shock and hemorrhage. A badly injured person or a person having history of major operation will have a low BP if untreated. The lost blood due to hemorrhage is replaced by whole blood. The blood volume reduced because of shock will be brought back to normal by giving saline or dextrose solution.
2. **Cardiac output:** The cardiac output depends on the volume of blood that returns to the heart by the veins. If the venous return is poor, the amount of blood is weak and the BP is low. If a person has to stand still for a long period of time, the venous return from the lower limbs is inhibited because of gravity and lack of exercise so the heartbeat weakens, the BP falls, which results in a faint.
3. **Elasticity of the large arteries:** The elasticity maintains the continuous flow of the blood throughout the periphery of the body. As the arteries stretch and recoil, they push the blood into the smaller vessels. In the old age, the walls of these vessels get hardened so a greater pressure of the blood against the inelastic walls is required.
4. **Caliber of the small arterioles called peripheral resistance:** This is the state of slight contraction of the muscular walls of the arterioles, producing the resistance to the flow of blood. These vessel walls can dilate or contract, depending on the amount of blood required by the organ they supply. Heat cause vasodilatation in the skin and cold causes vasoconstriction. When the vessels are dilated, the pressure is lower, and when they are constricted, the pressure is greater.
5. **Arterial stiffness:** This occurs secondary to hypertension. It is general thickening and stiffening of arterial wall, also called as atherosclerosis.

Systemic Arterial Blood Pressure

The BP is because of the flow of blood from the left ventricle into the already full aorta.

Systolic Blood Pressure

It is the maximum pressure exerted on the artery walls during the heart contraction. The pressure is about 120 mm Hg when the blood from left ventricle enters into aorta.

Diastolic Blood Pressure

It is the minimal pressure exerted on the artery walls when the heart is resting. The pressure is about 80 mm Hg, which occurs during complete cardiac diastole.

Pulse Pressure

The pulse pressure is systolic BP minus diastolic BP, which varies with different time of a day, posture, gender, and age of the individual.

The BP is low during night compared to day, low in females when compared to males, BP increases with age secondary to the structural changes in the arteries like atherosclerosis and is associated with high-risk of having cardiovascular diseases. Blood pressure is measured by an instrument called sphygmomanometer. The normal range is 120/80 mm Hg.

Control of Blood Pressure

The BP is controlled by the homeostasis and regulated by the cardiovascular center located in medulla and pons. This cardiovascular center receives, integrates and coordinates the input from the baroreceptors, chemoreceptors and higher centers in the brain. The output of the cardiovascular center is through the autonomic nervous system to the heart and blood vessels, enabling the rapid response to change in blood pressure.

Baroreceptors

These are situated in the arch of aorta and carotid sinuses.

Functions

The baroreceptors are sensitive to stretch that increases or decreases the blood pressure. When the BP is increased, a signal is sent to activate cardiovascular center, the baroreceptors and 28 physiology chemoreceptors are stretched. This center responds by adjustment

Physiology

in output to the heart and blood vessels. The blood vessels become dilated, and stroke volume and the HR decrease, thereby decreasing the BP.

Chemoreceptors

These are the nerve endings situated in carotid and aortic bodies. They are primarily involved in control of respiration. These are sensitive to change in level of carbon dioxide, oxygen, and acidity of blood (pH).

Higher Centers of Brain

The stimulation of the higher centers of the brain is affected by the input of fear, anxiety, pain, anger, and emotional state, which brings changes in the BP. The hypothalamus controls the body temperature, which influences the cardiovascular center. This center responds by adjusting the diameter of the blood vessels in the skin. So the important mechanism is determining the heat loss and heat retention.

Normal blood pressure range values in infant, child and adult:
Infant: 65-95/30-60 mm Hg
Child: 85-120/50-80 mm Hg
Adult: 120-129/80-84 mm Hg

APPLIED ANATOMY

Hypotension: The condition with low blood pressure is called hypotension. The pressure is around 90/60 mm Hg. If the pressure drops quickly it is too dangerous and could damage tissues and organs of the body. Orthostatic hypotension or postural hypotension is a condition where blood pressure falls to low when the person is sitting up or stand. This condition is too dangerous too. Symptoms of hypotension are dizziness, cardiogenic shock. Conditions with hypotension are addition disease, sepsis, cardiogenic shock and hemorrhage.

Treatment: Drink more water as fluids increases blood volume and prevents dehydration

Prognosis: Low blood pressure is dangerous as less blood flows to the organs leading to heart attack, stroke and kidney failure leading to shock and death.

Hypertension: The condition with high blood pressure is called hypertension.
Grades of hypertension are:
Normal BP: 120 and 80 mm Hg
Elevated BP: 120-129 and > 80 mm Hg
Grade 1/ Stage 1 Hypertension: 130-139 or 80-89 mm Hg
Grade 2/ Stage 2 Hypertension: 140 or higher or 90 or higher mm Hg
Grade 3 /Hypertensive crisis: >180 and or >120 mm Hg
(Patient need to consult the doctor immediately)

Complications: Severe stage can lead to heart attack, stroke, kidney failure.

Treatment: Diet with less salt, daily exercise and medication with regular check up and frequent follow up under the guidance of physician.

THE COUGH REFLEX

Coughing is a protective reflex. Cough reflex has two components: sensory component and motor component, both function via vagus nerve. It is the most common feature of all respiratory disorders. This is the most common symptom of all respiratory disorders. The reflex occurs with a brief inspiration followed by that is closure of the glottis, contraction of the expiratory muscles (abdominals) resulting in the rise in intra-abdominal pressure or intrathoracic pressure. This forces the epiglottis to open and causes a rapid flow of the expired air to come out with sputum and if the long duration is seen then cough can be the symptom of bacterial and viral infection and if the same continues patient should visit the doctor. Cough can be dry or productive and the character varies according to disorder or disease.

Stimulus

The cough reflex is stimulated by the following—food, fluid, foreign bodies, cigarette smoking and pollutant.

Receptors

Cough reflex receptors are called lung irritant receptors. They have nerve supply from vagus nerve. The receptors are located in between respiratory epithelial cells and throughout the respiratory tract. The receptors in the large bronchi produce cough and the receptors in the small bronchi produced bronchoconstriction. Cough receptors are sensitive to chemical and mechanical stimuli, sulfur dioxide, or chlorine gas.

Pathology

The cough reflex is impaired because of following reasons: 1. Respiratory and abdominal muscle weakness occurs secondary to paralysis, surgery, muscle weakness, prolonged bed rest causing physical inactivity, injury to superior laryngeal nerve affecting reflex arc of cough reflex, foreign object lodged in laryngopharynx. All these causes weak and ineffective cough reflex due to interference with chest expansion which is limiting the intake of air helping for coughing.

Test

Inhaling the air with nebulizer.

Treatment

Cough suppressants for dry cough such as antihistamines. These expectorants bring mucus from lungs, bronchi, and trachea and physical therapy treatment called chest physical therapy.

The Chest Physical Therapy

Definition

The chest physical therapy is an airway clearance techniques performed to remove the secretions.

Technique

The chest physical therapy is divided as two programs. They are dependent program where physical therapist performs the technique and independent program where patient performs the program as part of home exercise program.

S. No.	Dependent program techniques	Independent program techniques
1.	Postural drainage	Active cycle of breathing techniques
2.	Percussion	PEP (positive expiratory pressure), e.g., Thera PEP
3.	Vibration	Airway oscillation device (flutter, Acapella)
4.	Airway clearance techniques like coughing, huffing	High frequency chest compression (HFCC), e.g., Vest system

Dependent Chest Physical Therapy

Postural drainage: This techniques is removal of secretion using gravity assisted position, e.g., Trendelenburg position.

Indications:
- Atelectasis
- Aspiration
- Increased pulmonary secretions

Technique: Explain the procedure to the patient and with patient consent, the patient is positioned in Trendelenburg position (head tipped down 15 to 18 degrees). Check for signs of intolerance. The techniques performed are percussion, vibration, airway clearance techniques. The duration for each position can be up to 20 minutes.

Percussion: This is the techniques performed using cupped hands rhythmically on the chest wall. This technique is performed for specialized area for 3 to 5 minutes.

The uses of postural drainage: Releases pulmonary secretions from walls of the airways to the lumen of the airways. The secretions can be enhanced effectively.

Indications:
- Prolonged bed rest
- Postoperative patients
- Stable ventilator patients

Contraindications:
- Pulmonary embolism
- Unstable angina
- Recent neuroimaging
- Fracture
- Osteoporosis

Precautions:
- Osteoporosis
- Decreased platelet count
- Flail chest
- Fracture ribs

Shaking: The patient is asked to take 5-7 deep inhalation, physical therapist places hands on the rib cage Trendenlenburg position.

Air way clearance techniques: Once secretions are mobilized using above passive techniques then patient is asked to start with airway clearance techniques. The techniques are:
- *Coughing:* The coughing is one of the easiest way of removing secretions but in patient with chronic pulmonary lung disease. Due to high intrathoracic pressure during coughing causes to closing of smaller airways. So huffing is performed for those patients instead of coughing.
- *Huffing:* Patient is asked to take a deep breath and rapidly contract abdominal muscles by forcefully saying HA HA HA.

Active cycle breathing techniques: The ACBT is an independent program where patient can perform as home exercise program to clear the secretions from the airways. The ACBT techniques are:
- Breathing control phase
- Thoracic expansion exercises
- Forced expiratory technique

Breathing control phase (BCP): In this phase the patient is asked to perform relaxed diaphragmatic breathing.

Indications:
- Chronic obstructive lung diseases
- Restrictive lung diseases

Position of patient: Semi-Fowler's position or semi-reclined position.

Technique: The patient is asked to perform inspiration and during expiration the patient puts gentle pressure by placing the hands on the subcostal angle of the thorax. The patient is asked to exhale against the resistance of physical therapist hands. The pressure is released during inspiration and the same technique is repeated. The progression of the same technique is performed in different positions like upright sitting and standing.

Uses:
- Improves gaseous exchange
- Increase ventilation
- Decreases work of breathing
- Improves chest wall mobility
- Facilitate relaxation

Thoracic expansion exercise (TEE): The patient is asked to perform deep respirations with 3 seconds hold after inspiration and followed by expiration.

Forced expiratory technique (FET): The patient performs 1 or 2 huffs. This techniques helps to move secretions from smaller to larger airway.

Oral airway oscillation devices: The devices used are flutter or Acapella. The patient inhales normally and exhales through the device for 10 breaths followed by this perform coughing or huffing.

Positive expiratory pressure (PEP): The PEP is of two types: low pressure PEP and high pressure PEP.

S. No.	Low pressure positive expiratory pressure	High pressure positive expiratory pressure
1.	Low pressure PEP is used at 10 to 20 cm H_2O measurement	High pressure PEP is used at 50 to 120 mm H_2O measurement
2.	Position of patient: Sitting	Position of patient: Sitting
3.	The patient inhales and exhales through the mask or mouth piece.	The patient inhales and exhales through the mask or mouth piece.

Contd...

Contd...

S. No.	Low pressure positive expiratory pressure	High pressure positive expiratory pressure
	Patient performs this for 10–20 minutes then removes mask and performs coughing or huffing	Patient performs this for 10–20 minutes then through the mask performs coughing or huffing
4.		High PEP is used for patients with unstable airways

High frequency chest wall oscillation (HFCWO): In this technique the patient wears the vest. The vest is filled with air. This increase the pressure until patient has sung fit of the Vest or decrease pressure. The frequency treatment time is 20 to 30 minutes.

BREATHING, LUNG COMPLIANCE, AND AIRWAY RESISTANCE

Breathing

Breathing is the regular inflation and deflation of the lung which maintains a steady concentration of atmospheric gases in the alveoli, i.e., the constant intake of oxygen and output of carbon dioxide.

Factors Affecting the Breathing

1. **Elasticity:** The loss of elasticity of the connective tissue in the lung necessitates forced expiration and increased effort on inspiration.
2. **Compliance:** Compliance is the measure of distensibility of the lungs, i.e., the effort required to inflate the alveoli. When compliance is low, the effort needed to inflate the lungs is greater than normal, e.g., in restricted lung disease, the elasticity is reduced or the presence of insufficient surfactant leads to decrease of lung compliance.
3. **Airflow resistance:** The airway resistance is increased in broncho-resistance. So more effort is required to inflate the lungs.

Disorders of breathing:
- Hypopnea and hypoventilation means shallow breathing
- Hyperpnea and hyperventilation means deep breathing

Lung Compliance

Definition

The lung compliance is the measure of the elasticity of the alveolar walls and is measured as the changes in the volume produced by the change in the unit pressure.

Alveoli with high compliance expand more than those with low compliance for a given pressure. The lung tissue that is stiffened by disease has a low compliance, and it is hard work for a patient to generate the forces to expand the lungs; therefore it reduces the use of ventilation. The lung compliance is decreased by stiff lungs or by a stiff chest wall called the restricted lung disease or kyphoscoliosis.

Lung compliance is also called pulmonary compliance. It is of two types:
1. **Static compliance:** It occurs with volume change with applied pressure.
2. **Dynamic compliance:** It occurs with actual air movement.

Factors Affecting the Compliance

1. Pulmonary tissue
2. Chest wall

Pulmonary tissue

The pulmonary tissue in turn has some factors that affect its function such as the following:
1. **Elastic fibers of the lung:** The elastic recoil opposes the stretching of the lung; hence, the reduction of the elastic coil causes a rise in compliance and vice versa.
2. **The surface tension within the alveoli:** The surfactant is the material present in the alveolus that reduces the surface tension exerted by the alveolar fluid. The surfactant is the mixture of phospholipid and the proteins. The type-II alveolar cells secrete this. In the newborn, the surfactant is less and the disease is called hyaline membrane disease or respiratory distress syndrome. The surfactant is produced only in the later stages of the fetal life. So there is great inspiratory difficulty as the compliance of the lung is very low, hence may lead to pulmonary edema.
3. **Interdependence**: Few of the adjacent alveoli start to collapse. The neighboring alveoli start pulling the collapsing alveoli and their collapse is opposed.

Chest wall

The chest wall is highly elastic and springs out. The disease of the chest wall causes a reduction of the compliance, e.g., ankylosing spondylitis and kyphoscoliosis.

Pathology

Low compliance

Stiffening of chest wall with high elastic recoil seen in conditions such as fibrosis.

High compliance
Pliable and low elastic recoil is seen in conditions such as emphysema and COPD.

Airway Resistance

The resistance given by the airways is called airway resistance. The place of the greatest airway resistance is in the upper respiratory tract where the total cross-sectional area is narrowest and airflow is most turbulent. The nasal route gives more resistance; a person breathes through the mouth when breathlessness or exercising because the resistance of the airflow is less. Airway distends on inspiration and compresses on expiration. The patient will have difficulty in breathing out than breathing in. On expiration, the resistance rises most steeply.

The airway resistance also increases in acute cases of asthma and in COPD because the airway is obstructed. The further obstruction and loss of the elastic recoil are caused in emphysema.

Airway resistance can be measured by using body plethysmography.

Factors affecting the airway resistance are:
1. **The phase of inspiration and expiration**: The intrapleural and the mediastinal pressure become negative, and increase in negativity leads to increase in bronchial diameter. The resistance to the airflow is normally low. During expiration, the intrapleural and mediastinal negativity decreases; therefore bronchial diameter gets reduced. The resistance to the airflow is high. During normal breathing, the expiration is approximately 1.4 times longer than the inspiration because the air requires greater time for the exit, e.g., the bronchial asthma is associated with bronchospasm, inspiration may not be difficult but expiration is very touch. So wheeze is heard during expiration.
2. **Tone of the bronchial muscle**: This is associated with bronchospasm and bronchoconstriction. The B2 adrenergic stimulation causes powerful relaxation so diminishes airway resistance. Histamine, proteoglycans, irritant fumes, and channel blockers cause bronchospasm. Bronchoconstriction is caused by exposure to irritant gases, cigarette smoking. This is also seen in the case of bronchial asthma.
3. **The density of the air**: If the density of the inspired air is high the resistant to airway flow increases and vice versa.

Pathology

1. **Asthma attack:** Increase airway resistance causes constriction of airways.
2. **Emphysema:** Increased airway resistance and constriction of airways.

THE DIFFUSION, VENTILATION, AND PERFUSION

Diffusion

The exchange of gases occurs when the difference in partial pressure exists across the semipermeable membrane. The diffusion occurs in both gaseous and liquid states, leading to equilibrium. The gases move by diffusion from the higher concentrations to the lower concentration until equilibrium is established. In the peripheral airways, the gaseous exchange occurs by gaseous diffusion between the respiratory bronchioles and the alveolar walls. The gases then diffuse through the membrane and fluid and reach hemoglobin. This occurs by equalizing the oxygen tension. And the red cells have traversed only one-third of the way and the carbon oxide diffuse 20 times easily.

The diffusion capacity is defined as a measure of diffusing oxygen and carbon dioxide from lungs to blood. The diffusion capacity helps to diagnose the severity of lung diseases like restrictive and obstructive lung diseases and before surgery to know about the prognosis.

Three reasons for diffusion capacity testing are:
1. To know if the treatment is improving or worsening the lung condition.
2. To know the severity of emphysema.
3. To know patient with lung cancer if he/she can tolerate the surgery.

Normal range of diffusion capacity:
Males: 80–120%
Females: 76–120%.

Values of the Diffusion

1. Efficiency of the ventilation
2. Ventilation and perfusion ratio
3. Oxygen-carrying capacity
4. Efficiency of the circulation

5. Metabolic rate
6. Acidity or alkalinity of the blood

Blood gas measurement gives an indication of ventilation, gas exchange, and the acid-base state.

The PaO_2: This is the partial pressure of oxygen in arterial blood. It is the amount of oxygen dissolved in plasma. The normal value is 80-100 mm Hg or 11-14 kPa.

The $PaCO_2$: This is the partial pressure of carbon dioxide. The normal value is 35-45 mm Hg or 4.7-6.0 kPa.

Partial pressure of oxygen is only 3% of oxygen dissolved in plasma and reflects the pressure needed to push it from air to blood and blood to tissue cells.

The SaO_2 is the extent to which the hemoglobin is saturated with oxygen and represents the capacity of blood to carry oxygen. Normal value is 95-98%. The SaO_2 describes the 97% of oxygen that is bound to hemoglobin. An anemic person will have normal SaO_2 but delivers a subnormal load of oxygen.

The ventilation, diffusion, and perfusion occur in sequence. The gas exchange occurs at tissue level to complete the process of respiration. The oxygen transport depends on the cardiac output and oxygen content of the blood. The oxygen delivery and utilization depend upon local perfusion, metabolic rate, and oxygen demand.

Testing: The lung diffusion testing detects the flow of oxygen and carbon dioxide in between lungs and blood. The name of the test is called DLCO (diffusing capacity of the lung for CO) test.

Indication: Lung diseases.

Goal: To improve lung functioning.

Test:
Normal: 75-140%
Mild reduction in lung function: 60-70%
Severe reduction in lung function: <40%

Abnormal values are seen in conditions such as asthma, emphysema, foreign body, pulmonary embolism, lung hemorrhage, arterial blood flow issues, and pulmonary hypertension.

Clinical Application

- Hypoxia: This is decreased cardiac output, decreased oxygen-carrying capacity of the blood and increased oxygen needs.

- Hypoxemia: This is caused because of hypoventilation, diffusion abnormality, wasted perfusion, and ventilation.
- Hypoventilation: The ventilation decreases, the carbon dioxide accumulates, and partial pressure of carbon dioxide rises.
- Diffusion abnormalities: This is related to oxygen.

The Ventilation—Perfusion and their Interrelationship

Ventilation

Definition
The ventilation is the supply of oxygen through the lungs. It occurs by RCs in medulla oblongata and pons of brain stem.

Alveolar ventilation: This is the volume of air that moves into and out of the alveoli per minute. This is equal to tidal volume minus the anatomical dead space multiplied by respiratory rate. (TV − anatomical dead space) multiplied by respiratory rate = (500–150) mL multiplied by 15/min = 5.25 L/min.

Tidal volume
The volume of air breathed in and out during a quiet respiration. It is about 500 mL. About 150 mL of this volume amount remains in the dead space in tracheobronchial tree where no gaseous exchange occurs. The rest 350 mL is present in the alveoli, alveolar duct where gaseous exchange occurs. This is about 350 mL called alveolar ventilation.

Example: The respiratory rate is about 14/min, tidal volume is 500 mL. The total ventilation rate or ventilation per minute or respiratory minute volume is about 500 multiplied by 14 mL/min = 7 L/min. The dead space around 150 mL then the alveolar ventilation is 500 − 150 mL multiplied 14/min = 4.9 L/min.

Most of the dead space ventilation is made up of anatomical dead space that represents the air in the conducting passages that is last in and first out this does not reach the alveoli. The alveolar dead space represents the air that reaches the alveoli but not the blood and is minimal in normal lungs. The sum of anatomical and alveolar dead space is called physiological dead space.

The alveoli in upper regions are more inflated because the lung hanging in the frame of the chest exerts expanding stress. Alveoli in lower regions are more squashed because there is less lung hanging down below them. The sponge-like properties of the lung mean ventilation is greater in the poorly expanded dependent regions where there is more potential to expand.

In the horizontal position, the excursion of the dependent portion of the diaphragm is twice that of the upper portion because the lower fibers are more stretched by the abdominal pressure and therefore contract from a position of mechanical advantage.

The rapid shallow breathing means that more tidal volume, since the same air is going in and out more often. Deep breathing increases lung compliance by stretching alveoli and encouraging surfactant production. The resistance between adjacent lung segments through collateral channels decreases with increased lung volume thus improving the distribution of ventilation.

Perfusion

The perfusion is also required for gaseous exchange in the lung. The pulmonary circulation is a low resistance system and has the unusual ability to further reduce its resistance in response to a rise in pressure by increasing the caliber of capillaries and recruiting others that are closed.

Such a low-pressure system is very responsive to gravity, so there is a steep perfusion gradient from top to the bottom of the lung. In the base of the upright lung, the greater volume of blood leads to airway closure. In the apex, perfusion is minimal because the arterial pressure can't overcome alveolar pressure. These delicate vessels collapse in upper lung if the balance is disturbed.

Perfusion becomes more evenly distributed when a person lies own or takes exercise. It is more unevenly distributed in people with COPD.

Ventilation–Perfusion Ratio

Definition

The ventilation perfusion is the ratio of the alveolar ventilation and the amount of blood that perfuses the alveoli.

V = ventilation: air reaching alveoli
P = perfusion: blood reaching alveoli
V/Q: amount of air reaching alveoli per minute/amount of blood reaching the alveoli per minute
VPR = VA/Q
VA = alveolar ventilation
Q = perfusion or the blood flow

Normal values

Alveolar ventilation = 4,200 mL/min
Perfusion = 5,000 mL/min

VPR = 4,200/5,000 = 0.84

Measurement: by V/P scan
V/P mismatch is the type of respiratory failure
1 L of blood holds 200 mL of oxygen
1 L of blood holds 210 mL of oxygen
V:P ratio is 0.95
The lung superior part is called apex of lung and inferior part is called base of lung.
Apex of lungs: high V/Q ratio
Base of lungs: lower V/Q ratio

Significance

The significance of ventilation–perfusion ratio is gaseous exchange.
Note: This is affected by any change of ventilation and perfusion.

Variation
1. **Physiological variation:**
   a. The ratio increases with the increase in ventilation and no change in perfusion.
   b. The ratio decreases if perfusion increases without any change in ventilation.
   c. In sitting position, there is a reduction in perfusion and ventilation in the upper part of the lung than the lower part.
   d. The reduction in perfusion is more than a reduction in ventilation so VPR increases three times.
   e. The VPR ratio decreases in the base of the lung because of low V/Q ratio.
   f. The physiological shunt occurs because a part of blood does not get oxygenated.
2. **Pathological variation:** In COPD such as emphysema, the ventilation is affected because of the obstruction and destruction of the alveolar membrane. So VPR is drastically decreased.

Perfusion

Exchange at tissue level
Diffusion: Exchange between capillaries and alveoli
Ventilation: Exchange in and out of the lungs
Hypoxia: Perfusion problems
Hypoxemia: Diffusion problems
   Shunt is the area with no ventilation but with perfusion only. So V/Q is ZERO.
   Dead space is the area with ventilation and no perfusion. So V/Q is undefined.

A lower V/Q ratio impairs pulmonary gas exchanges and low PaO_2, e.g., chronic bronchitis and acute pulmonary edema.

A high V/Q ratio decreases $PaCO_2$ and increases PaO_2 causes tachypnea and dyspnea, e.g., pulmonary embolism and emphysema.

Abnormalities of ventilation perfusion ratio V/Q defects or total lung ventilation perfusion ratio defects. These are the areas of lung either receive oxygen or no blood flow or receive blood flow and no oxygen. The normal lung ventilation/perfusion ratio is 0.8. The alveolar ventilation and pulmonary blood flow are equal. The ratio can be detected by ventilation perfusion scan or lung scintigraphy conditions affected by ventilation: perfusion ratio are:

S. No.	Condition	Ventilation	Perfusion	Physical therapy treatment
1.	Pulmonary embolism	Normal	Decreases causing hypoxemia	Oxygen therapy breathing exercises
2.	Asthma	Abnormal causes atelectasis	Normal	Breathing exercises positioning
3.	Pneumonia	Abnormal	Abnormal	Oxygen therapy breathing exercises positioning

THE ENERGY EXPENDITURE

The human body requires the energy to support normal function, physical activities, and growth of a repair of damaged tissue. The energy is provided by oxidation of dietary fat, protein, carbohydrate, and alcohol. A small part of energy is by breakdown of animal's own tissue. The protein energy of food provides kinetic energy of the body in the form of heat and work. The unit of energy is calorie. Calorie is the amount of heat required to the temperature of 1 g of water by 1°C. One kilocalorie is equal to 4.2 kJ.

Measurement of Energy Values of Food

The foodstuffs such as carbohydrates, fat, and protein on combustion by oxygen produce heat. The heat is measured by the bomb calorimeter.
1 g of carbohydrates = 4 kcal
1 g of proteins = 4 kcal
1 g of fat = 9 kcal

Energy Expenditure in Healthy Adults

This depends on the three factors:
1. Body size

2. Physical activities:
   a. Light activities (sedentary) such as office work with mechanical gadgets
   b. Moderate activities such as printing, housewife without mechanical gadgets
   c. Heavy activities such as agriculture workers, unskilled laborers
3. Age.

Energy Expenditure Determined by Three Factors

1. Basal metabolic rate or BMR/basal energy expenditure or BEE/resting metabolic rate: It is the amount of energy the body requires at rest. This is the energy required to maintain the basic physiological function. BMR is 60–75% of total energy expenditure.
2. Thermogenesis or thermic effect of food: It is the amount of energy expanded during and following the ingestion of the food.
3. Physical activity: This has a major implication on the energy expenditure.

The energy expenditure with various physical activities are done during sitting, standing, walking, etc.

Body mass index = weight in kilograms/height in square meters.

Physical therapy management for energy conservation:

S. No.	Aims of physical therapy	Goals of physical therapy
1.	Teach activity pacing	Breathing in during rest and breath out and perform activities like activities of daily living, walking, stair climbing Avoid prolonged standing, squatting, stooping
2.	Energy conservation techniques	Frequent rest breaks Distribution of work Sitting and performing activities, stopping when feeling fatigue
3.	Minimize muscle fatigue	Patients education

Basal Metabolism

The basic amount of energy spent to survive is called basal metabolism, e.g. sleeping, breathing, maintain body temperature, etc.

Factors

1. **Surface area:** The larger is the surface area, the greater is the BMR.
2. **Age:** The children have larger BMR than adults.
3. **Sex:** Males have higher BMR than adults.

4. **Emotion:** The BMR increases in the emotional stress.
5. **BMR:** This is normal in starvation, undernutrition, hypothalamic disorders, Addison's disease and below normal in fever, diabetes, leukemia, and polycythemia.

Determination of Energy Metabolism

Principles

1. Measuring the volume of expired air during work for a fixed period of 5-10 minutes
2. Collection of a sample of expired air or the analysis of oxygen and carbon dioxide contents
3. Calculation of oxygen consumption, carbon dioxide output, and respiratory quotient
4. Calculation of energy output from respiratory quotient and oxygen consumption

Measurement

1. **Douglas bag:** This is the lab test performed and the bag is made of rubber. The capacity of the bag is 100 liters and the patient is asked to breath into the bag for a period of 5 to 6 minutes. The air in the bag is then measured using a gas meter and a sample taken for the analysis of oxygen and carbon dioxide.
2. **Max–Planck respirometer:** The instrument is portable. This works simultaneously by measuring directly the volume of the expired air and passing a small quantity into the rubber bladder attached to it. The air is analyzed for carbon dioxide and oxygen. Respiratory quotient is found as volume of carbon dioxide produced/volume of the oxygen consumed.

Basic Metabolic Rate (BMR) and Physical Therapy Management

The physical therapy management focusses on BMR, total daily calorie consumption and various methods for weight management and staying fit and healthy.

The BMR is the amount of calories an individual will burn in one day at rest.

To know the total daily energy expenditure and physical activity during the weak are calculated. To maintain healthy weight the calorie consumption should not exceed calories burn each day.

Basic metabolic rate and total daily energy expenditure. The following table explains in details:

S. No.	Activity level	Exercise level	Example
1.	Sedentary	Little or no exercise	Desk job
2.	Lightly active	Light sports	Playing 1–3 days sports
3.	Moderate active	Moderate exercise	Playing 3–5 days sports
4.	Very active	Hard exercise	Playing 6–7 days sports
5.	Extra active	Hard daily exercise	Marathon

Basal Metabolic Rate:

S. No.	BMI	Status
1.	Below 18.5	Underweight
2.	BMI 18.5–24.9	Normal weight
3.	BMI 25.0–29.9	Over weight
4.	BMI 30	Obesity
5.	BMI 40	Morbid obesity

Weight loss: The weight loss can be seen when there is balance between eating less calories and burn more calories. There are 3500 calories in one pound of stored body fat. To loose one pound we need deficits of 3500 calories.

Weight training: This is also called resistance training. This increase lean body mass.

Tissues of body: There are two tissues in the body. They are fat tissue and muscle. The muscle has high calorie consumption for performing functions like regulates body temperature, gaseous exchange, restore nutrients and circulate blood. So increase metabolic rate and decrease body fat. So more calories are burn when muscle mass is increased even sitting at desk, sleeping and relaxing.

Exercise to increase energy expenditure: The exercise should be performed 6 to 7 days a week. The weight management includes diet, exercises, balance calorie consumption, staying fit and healthy.

Avoid low calorie diet: It decreases metabolic rate because strict diet causes thyroid not working properly. Metabolic slow, lean body mass is lost. The ideal weight can be reached by keeping small calorie deficit and increased activity level in the week. The weight loss can be tracked using BMI. It is a screening tool to diagnose body fat and health risk.

PULMONARY FUNCTION ASSESSMENT

Assessment of the Pulmonary Patient

1. Introduction
2. Database
    a. Ward reports and meetings
    b. Notes and charts
3. Subjective assessment
    a. Symptoms
    b. Functional limitations
4. Observation
    a. Apparatus
    b. Sputum
    c. General appearance
    d. Color
    e. Hands
5. Edema
    a. Chest shape
    b. Breathing rate
    c. Breathing pattern
    d. Jugular venous pressure
6. Palpation
    a. Abdomen
    b. Chest expansion
    c. Percussion note
    d. Hydration
    e. Trachea
7. Auscultation
    a. Technique
    b. Breath sounds
    c. Added sounds
    d. Voice sounds
8. Exercise tolerance
9. Chest X-ray
10. Pulmonary function test

Introduction

The patient assessment is very important because evaluating the patient helps to create physical therapy aims and goals to be achieved by the patient in order to get back to the prior level of functioning. So the evaluation is done in quiet environment to make patient feel

comfortable and patient is able to express themselves. The plan of action is as follows:
1. Assess the patient
2. Identify problems
3. Correlate these with the patient's expectations
4. Formulate goals with the patient
5. Plan management and its time frame
6. Treatment
7. Reassess
8. Modify the management plan according to on-going assessment
9. Reviews

Database

Ward reports and meetings
The physiotherapist should take referrals from the medical staff and the nursing staff and should plan out physiotherapy treatment required, and the changes in the patient conditions can be explained and a note can be written in the case sheet.

Notes and charts
The details required before starting the physiotherapy treatment are as follows:
1. History of vertigo or light-headedness
2. Swallowing difficulty or tendency to aspirate
3. Tendency to bleed
4. Social history
5. Arthritis
6. Elevated white cell count, recent infection
7. Recent cardiopulmonary resuscitation (need an X-ray examination in case of aspiration or fracture)
8. Bony metastasis
9. Steroid therapy
10. Radiotherapy over chest (8, 9, 10 are contraindicated for percussion or vibrations over the ribs)
11. Temperature chart at every check (infection or atelectasis)
12. Drug therapy
13. Oxygen therapy
14. Fluid balance
15. Dehydration
16. Sputum retention
17. Blood pressure
18. Heart rate

Subjective Assessment

Symptoms
1. How long have symptoms been troublesome?
2. Are the symptoms better or worse?
3. What are the aggravating ad relieving factors?
4. Chest disease symptoms such as
   a. Wheeze (tightness of the chest on breathing out, noisy breathing, and the aggravating factors such as exertion and other factors)
   b. Pain can be as chest pain which can be sharp and stabbing as pleuritic type pain, in pleurisy, and severe pain on deep breathing and coughing. Paroxysmal suffocating pain due to myocardial ischemia pneumonia, spontaneous pneumothorax and pulmonary embolism, angina pectoris, and raw central chest pain worse on coughing caused by tracheitis with upper respiratory tract infection.
   c. Breathlessness:
      i. How does your condition affect your lungs?
      ii. Do you smoke? How many times? Its effects on health?
      iii. Do you become tired? Is it exhausting to clear your chest? How about exercise every day?
      iv. How are your appetite, its effects, and types of food you take?
      v. Do you have any problems of facing constipation and seeking its solution?
      vi. Are you under prescription of inhalers or tablets and their use?
      vii. Is oxygen available at home, what flow rate you use? Time of use and how does it help you?
      viii. Is breathlessness becoming barrier to your activities of daily living?
      ix. How breathless are you now (no breathlessness or very severe breathlessness) and feeling of it (worried, frustrated, embarrassed, frightened, and depressed)?
      x. How far can you walk, transport?
   d. Cough with or without sputum:
      i. How did cough start?
      ii. How is sputum like?
      iii. How is the quality and quantity?
      iv. Is there blood also?
      v. Does the cough make you awake?
      vi. Is this also with eating and drinking?

Functional limitation
1. Activities of daily living
2. Finance
3. Employment
4. Housing
5. Daily exercise
6. Employment
7. Number of stairs at workplace or home
8. Environment dusty, smoky?
9. Habits such as smoking, living alone, and eating well
10. Are there any difficulties to shop, bathe, and dress?
11. Patient's opinion on disease?
12. Does patient have anxiety, depression, fatigue, frustration, embarrassment, and restricted social function?

Observation

1. Breathing rate or respiratory rate: It is number of breaths per min. This depends on ventilation, i.e. amount of air in and out of lungs. If the rate decreases then it is the first sign of deterioration. It is 12–20 breaths per minute.
2. Breathing pattern: It is assessment of breathing rate. The following are assessed: Ratio of inspiration to expiration. The normal is 2:1, the sequence of inspiration and expiration during chest wall movement and accessory muscle use.

Apparatus
Is the patient is on oxygen? If so how many liters, check if via nasal cannula, if patient is on Trach (it is a passage provided through patient's trachea called tracheostomy where patient breaths through plastic tube provided in the opening and this procedure is performed when patient's normal use of nose and mouth is reduced or blocked for breathing) and ventilator (this a machine that helps to breath). Check the patient for other drains and drips.

Sputum
1. **Pulmonary edema:** The patient will have white or pink color and frothy serous secretions.
2. **Chronic bronchitis:** The patient will have raw egg white sticky gray mucoid sputum.
3. **Asthma:** The patient will have tenacious, mucoid sputum, with thick plugs, excess eosinophils.
4. **Pseudomonas infection:** The patient will have foul-smelling green sputum.

5. Bronchiectasis, tuberculosis, mitral stenosis, pulmonary carcinoma lung contusion, and tracheal suction cause hemoptysis, and the vomit consists of blood and is bright red color blood.
6. **Hematemesis:** This condition is vomiting of stomach contents mixed with blood and is dark red in color or regurgitation of blood only and term melena is digested blood passed per rectum.

General appearance
The patient is assessed for level of consciousness, interaction, looking well/pale, active/agitated, lethargic, sweating/labored breathing, overall posture and movement.

Color
1. **Pallor:** Pallor is the paleness of the skin caused by anemia. Anemia is decrease in oxyhemoglobin level seen in palms and face.
2. **Plethoric appearance:** Excess red blood cells in blood called polycythemia.
3. **Cyanosis:** Bluish coloration caused by unsaturated hemoglobin in the blood because of heart or lung disease. This is of two types central cyanosis appears on the tongue and lips when partial pressure of oxygen becomes below 50 or 60 mm Hg where normal partial pressure of O_2 is 94–100% or mm Hg.

Peripheral cyanosis occurs at the fingers, toes, and ear lobes which signifies the problem of blood circulation.

Hands
1. **Clubbing:** This is seen in heart and lung disorder, bronchial asthma, and increased perfusion.
2. Hands are warm from peripheral vasodilatation. Tremor suggests carbon dioxide retention.
3. Wasting of the hand muscles is associated with recent malnutrition.

Edema

Accumulation at the ankles or sacral region depends on posture. In the respiratory patient, it implies an inadequate venous return to the heart and associated with the heart failure and COPD.

Chest shape
The chest shape can be assessed based on the following categories:
1. Aging
2. Kyphosis
3. COPD (ribs held horizontal position and loss of elastic recoil)
4. Scoliosis

5. Sternal deformities:
   a. Pigeon chest or pectus carinatum
   b. Barrel chest or pectus excavatum

Breathing rate
1. HR is increased because of lung/heart disease/pain/anxiety/anemia/fatigue.
2. Sudden increase in HR because of pulmonary edema, pulmonary embolus, spontaneous pneumothorax.
3. Decrease in HR is because of drug overdose, brain damage, and diabetic coma and exhaustion.

Breathing pattern
This shows lung or chest wall pathology, dyspnea, or neurological defect.

There are three types of breathing:
1. Cheyne-Stokes breathing
2. Labored breathing
3. Paradoxical breathing

Jugular venous pressure
The internal jugular vein pressure indicates the raised pressure in the right ventricle and vein will engorged visible above clavicle in conditions such as COPD.

S. No.	Condition	Palpation	Percussion	Breath sounds	Added sounds	Voice sounds
1.	Consolidation	Normal	Dull	Bronchial breathing	–	Increased
2.	Pneumothorax	Decreased	Hyper resonant	Decreased	–	Decreased
3.	Pleural effusion	Decreased	Dull	Decreased		Decreased
4.	Acute asthma	Hyper-inflated chest	Hyper resonant	Silent chest	Expiratory wheeze	Normal
5.	Emphysema	Pursed lip Breathing	Hyper resonant	Blood supply decreased	–	Decreased
6.	Chronic bronchitis	Barrel chest	Resonant	Normal	Wheeze	Normal
7.	Bronchiectasis	Normal	Resonant	Normal	Inspiratory, Expiratory crackles	Normal

Contd...

Contd...

S. No.	Condition	Palpation	Percussion	Breath sounds	Added sounds	Voice sounds
8.	Pulmonary edema	Normal	Resonant	Normal	Wheeze	Normal
9.	Interstitial lung disease	Normal	Resonant	Normal	End inspiratory-crackles	Normal
10.	Fibrosis	Expansion decreased on affected side	Dull over affected area	Normal	Localized end-inspiratory crackles	Normal

Exercise Tolerance

The exercise tolerance can be estimated by the subjected assessment of walking to the shop and patients' walking distance is calculated and objective assessment is calculated by 6-minute walk or walking upstairs. This assessment gives an idea about patient's daily life, gait, and fatigue.

Chest X-ray/Radiograph

The radiograph provides a unique insight into the state of the lungs and the chest wall to diagnose conditions affecting the chest, its contents, and nearby structures. The posterior–anterior view makes an optimum view of the lungs because the patient takes a deep breath from the standing position with shoulders abducted resulting in a low diaphragm and scapula held clear of the film. For the less mobile patient anterior view is taken. The film is partly obscured by the scapula, raised diaphragm, and the magnified heart.

Pulmonary Function Tests

The pulmonary function tests measure the lung function that can distinguish restrictive from the obstructive disorders.

Indications:
The indications of pulmonary function tests are as follows:
a. To diagnose the lung diseases like bronchitis, asthma and emphysema.
b. To know level of exposure to chemical at work and assess the lung function.
c. To Assess the causes of shortness of breath.

The air in the lung is classified into two divisions:
1. **Lung volumes:** The lung volumes are classified as follows:
   a. *Tidal volume (TV):* The volume of the air breathed in and out in a single normal quit respiration is called tidal volume. It is about 500 mL.
   b. *Inspiratory reserve volume (IRV):* The additional amount of the air inspired forcefully after the end of the normal inspiration is called inspiratory reserved volume. It is about 3,300 mL or 3.3 L.
   c. *Expiratory reserve volume (ERV):* The additional amount of the air that can be expired out forcefully after normal expiration is called expiratory reserve volume. The normal value is 1,000 mL or 1 L.
   d. *Residual volume (RV):* The amount of the air remaining in the lung even after the forced expiration is called residual volume. The normal value is 1,200 mL or 1.2 L.

   Importance:
   Residual volume is the amount of the air left in the lungs after expiratory reserve volume is expired. So there is always air left in the lung. So there is gaseous exchange happening in between the breaths. So residual volume air mixes with newly inhaled oxygenated air and gaseous exchange occurs. Residual volume also helps for preventing large fluctuations with oxygen and carbon dioxide gases exchange.

2. **Lung capacities:** The lung capacities include two or more primary volumes.
   They are:
   a. *Inspiratory capacity (IC):* This is the maximum volume of air inspired starting from end expiratory position. Its value is 3,800 mL (IC = TV + IRV = 500 + 3,300 = 3,800).
   b. *Vital capacity (VC):* This is the maximum amount of the air that can be expelled out forcefully after a maximal deep inspiration. Its value is 4,800 mL (VC = IRV + TV + ERV = 3,300 + 500 + 1,000 = 4,800 mL).
   c. *Functional residual capacity (FRC):* This is the volume of the air remaining in the lungs after normal expiration. Its value is 2,200 mL (FRC + ERV + RV = 1,000 + 1,200 = 2,200 mL).
   d. *Total lung capacity (TLC):* This is the amount of the air present in the lungs after a deep inspiration. It includes all the volumes. Its value is TLC = IRV + TV + ERV + RV = 3,300 + 500 + 1,000 + 1,200 = 6,000 mL.

Forced expiratory flow
A peak flow meter provides a quick and simple indication of airway obstruction. The test is performed thrice and the best of three is taken with rest in between.

Suggestions to the patient
1. The patient is asked to avoid tight clothes.
2. No to have a heavy meal before the test.
3. Do not smoke.
4. Giving the explanation and perform the technique of the test.
5. If the first reading is taken in one position, other two should be taken in the same position.
6. The physiotherapist should demonstrate the technique with mouthpiece.
7. The patient should hold the mouthpiece tightly.
8. The patient should take a deep breath until the lungs are completely full then blow short and sharp and as hard as possible.

Importance of the test
1. This test is very important with patients with unstable asthma because lung function can decline to 50-60% of normal before symptoms are noticeable.
2. This is useful in the chronic asthma to determine the right drug.
3. To evaluate ventilation by assessing the factors affecting the movement of gas in and out of the lungs.
4. To guide for the diagnosis, treatment plan, and prognosis.
5. To help therapist to plan for therapeutic goals, appropriate intervention according to the pulmonary problems, identify the permanent respiratory impairment and treatment plan.

Guidelines
1. The pulmonary function tests evaluate airway responsivity, ventilatory regulation, and ventilatory mechanics.
2. The pulmonary function tests allow the effect of hypoxia and hypercapnia.
3. The pulmonary function tests help in the assessment of ventilatory mechanics which is measurement of lung volumes occur in restrictive pulmonary diseases such as pneumonia, interstitial lung disease, pleural effusion, pleurisy, pneumonia, and there is decrease of forced flow rates in obstructive lung disease such as chronic bronchitis, emphysema, asthma, bronchiectasis, and cystic fibrosis.
4. The assessment of the ventilatory mechanics also permits evaluation of the effectiveness of physiotherapy.

5. The pulmonary function tests helps to find out the general progress of the disease process.
6. The pulmonary function tests helps in the determination of the pulmonary impairment.

Tests Performed by Physical Therapist

A rough estimation of the airway obstruction can be made by asking the patient to blow out a lighted match held 6 in. from the mouth and if the patient fails to do then this suggests an FEV1 of less than 1 L.

Measurement of the Pulmonary Function

The measurement of pulmonary function can be done by the following tests:
1. Spirometer test
2. Gas transfer test
3. Exercise testing
4. Quantitative perfusion/ventilation scanning test
5. Six-minute walk test
6. Stair climbing test.

Spirometer
The method by which the lung volumes and capacities are measured is called spirometry. The simple instrument used for this purpose is called spirometer. The modified spirometer is known as respirometer. The spirometer can be used only for a single breath. The repeated cycles of respiration cannot be recorded by using the spirometer because the carbon dioxide accumulated in the spirometer cannot be removed and oxygen or fresh air cannot be provided to the subject.

Respirometer
This is the modified spirometer. This has the facility of removing the carbon dioxide and supply of the oxygen. The carbon dioxide is removed by placing soda lime inside the instrument. The oxygen is supplied to the instrument from the oxygen cylinder by a suitable valve system.

Spirogram
The record of the lung volumes and capacities using spirometer or respirometer is called spirogram. The downward deflection of the spirogram indicates expiration and the upward curve denotes inspiration.

Computerized spirometer

This is a solid-state electronic equipment. The subject has to respire to a sophisticated transducer, which is connected to the instrument by means of a cable.

The residual volume, functional residual capacity, and the total lung capacity are measured by the nitrogen washout technique and helium dilution technique, not with the spirometry.

Helium Dilution Technique

1. **Functional residual capacity**: The respirometer is filled with the air containing a known quantity of helium. Initially, the subject breaths normally, then after the end of the expiration, the subject breathes from the respirometer. The helium from the respirometer enters the lungs and starts mixing with the air in lungs. After few minutes of breathing, the concentration of helium in the respirometer becomes equal to the concentration of helium in the lungs of the subject. This is called the equilibrium of helium. After this between respirometer and lung, the concentration of helium in respirometer is determined.
   $FRC = V(C_1-C_2)/C_2$
   C_1: Initial concentration of helium in the respirometer
   C_2: Final concentration of the helium in the respirometer
   V: Initial volume of air in the respirometer
   Example: $V = 5,000$ mL, $C_1 = 15\%$, $C_2 = 10\%$
2. **Residual volume:** The subject should start breathing from the respirometer after forced expiration.

Nitrogen Washout Method

The concentration of nitrogen in the air is 80%. So the total quantity of nitrogen in the lungs is measured so that the amount of air in the lungs can be calculated.

1. **Functional residual capacity:** The subject is asked to breathe normally. After the end of the normal expiration, the subject inspires pure oxygen through a valve and expires into a Douglas bag. This procedure is repeated for 6–7 minutes till the nitrogen in lungs is displaced by oxygen. The nitrogen comes to the Douglas bag.
   The FRC is calculated as:
   a. Volume of air collected in Douglas bag
   b. Concentration of nitrogen in the Douglas bag
   $FRC = C_1$ multiply V/C_2

V = Volume of air collected = 40,000 mL
C_1 = Concentration of nitrogen in the collected air = 50%
C_2 = Normal concentration of nitrogen in the air = 80%
FRC = 2,500 mL

2. **Residual volume:** The subject starts inhaling pure oxygen after the end of the forceful expiration.
3. **Gas transfer tests/TLCO testing, transfer factor/diffusion capacity:** This test gives information about how much oxygen is breath in through nose and how much carbon dioxide is breathe out from the mouth. The test is performed as follows. Ask the patient to hold the breath and breath in and out into a mouth piece.
4. **Exercise testing:** This test measures exercise capacity of the patient and evaluates both cardiac and respiratory system. This test is done before the patient undergoes surgery as a positive outcome of prognosis.
5. **Quantitative perfusion/ventilation scanning:** This test estimates the function of each lobe, region and overall lung performance. So this test is used to predict the prognosis after lung surgeries like pneumonectomy, lobectomy and lung resection.
6. **Six-minute walk:** This is the test where patient is asked to walk for 6 minutes. This test is a part of preoperative evaluation done for thoracic surgery to know the prognosis of uncomplicated post-operative recovery.
7. **Stair climbing:** This test is one of the exercise tolerance test where the patient is asked to ascend and descend stairs as a part of post surgery prognosis.

Clinical Application for Above Tests

1. For preoperative evaluation
2. For the diagnosis of the functional pulmonary disorders
3. Obstructive ventilatory disorders such as chronic bronchitis, emphysema, asthma, cystic fibrosis, and bronchiectasis
4. Restrictive ventilatory disorders such as fibrosing alveolitis, interstitial pneumonitis, and sarcoidosis, and chest wall deformities.

Assessment for Chronic Obstructive Pulmonary Disease

Chronic obstructive pulmonary disease (COPD) is a group of lung conditions where patient will have difficulty of breathing secondary to inflammation of lungs. Physical therapy rehabilitation will help to improve the following. They are:

1. The quality of life
2. Exercise capacity
3. Overall strength

The risk factors are:
- Pollutants both indoor and outdoor
- Smoking
- Inhaling toxic substances
- Respiratory problems during early childhood or prenatal stages

Common Types of Chronic Obstructive Pulmonary Disease

1. Emphysema: Alveoli are damaged causes dyspnea and chronic cough.
2. Chronic bronchitis: Chronic inflammation of bronchi causes cough, sputum, and mucus for 3 months per year and 2 consecutive years.

Clinical Features

1. Increased risk of falls secondary to balance problems
2. Weakness in arms and legs
3. Weight loss or gain because of nutritional problems
4. Depression
5. High BP.

Types

The COPD is classified into four major categories. They are:
1. Mild
2. Moderate
3. Severe
4. Very severe.

Assessment

1. History especially smoking history
2. Exposure to dust and chemicals
3. Medication history
4. Assessment of what makes symptoms worse and what helps in relieving them
5. Lung function test
6. Muscle strength test for arms and legs
7. Balance testing
8. Risk of falling
9. Exercise capacity by 6-minute walk test.

Physical therapy program is designed for 4 weeks which helps to:
1. Improve the quality of life
2. Decrease shortness of breath
3. Strategize for coping with COPD
4. Help with follow-up home program and resident able to participate at home, work and community.

Physical therapy intervention:
Once the pulmonary assessment is done and the patient is put on pulmonary rehabilitation program. The aims and plans are set according to the patients requirement with main goal to bringing the patient to perform activities of daily living.

S. No.	Aims of physical therapy	Goals of physical therapy
1.	To improve the upper body strength	Upper body ergometer help to improve strength and increase aerobic capacity and decreases shortness of breath
2.	To increase cardiovascular endurance	Using treadmill and NU step
3.		Strengthening exercises using resistance band and weights
4.	To perform Inspiratory muscle training	For decreasing shortness of breath and increases exercise capacity
5.	To decrease the shortness of breath and energy conservation	Pursed lip breathing and diaphragmatic breathing
6.	To decrease of fall risks	Static and dynamic balance training
7.	To decrease shortness of breath and leg fatigue	Walking endurance slowly increasing the distance and watching for symptoms like fatigue and shortness of breath
8.	Home exercise program	To continue all the above exercise as maintenance program and prevent returning of the symptoms and improving functional capacity and getting back to prior level of function

CARDIOVASCULAR STRESS TESTING

Principles

1. To evaluate coronary artery disease.
2. Exercise the patient on the treadmill and bicycle ergometer.
3. To record electrocardiograph (ECG) during and immediately after exercise.
4. To increase work till the patient attains the 140–170 desired level.

5. To make patient work till patient shows symptoms such as chest pain, giddiness, angina, and palpitation.
6. The test is effective with heart imaging with radioactive technique of thallium 99.
7. To increase cardiac output and stroke volume.
8. The sympathetic nervous system works maximum and the parasympathetic nervous system will be withdrawn and peripheral vasoconstriction occurs.
9. The adrenaline and the noradrenaline secretion causes a decrease in the blood supply.
10. The cardiac output increases 4–6 times than normal.

Contraindications

1. Unstable angina
2. Recent myocardial infarction
3. Untreated cardiac-arrhythmia
4. Congestive heart failure
5. Aortic stenosis
6. Cardiac myopathy
7. Acute myocarditis
8. Advanced atrioventricular (AV) block
9. Uncontrolled hypertension
10. Acute systemic illness

Procedure

The patient is asked to come with an empty stomach. No hot beverages should be taken. If the patient is a male who is undergoing the surgery, the chest should be shaved. The procedure should be explained. ECG should be taken initially before starting in resting position in sitting and lying position. Demonstrate the technique on treadmill and simultaneously record BP, ECG, and HR. The normal HR is 140–170 beats/min. Observe the patient if he/she has any giddiness, chest pain. Observe the changes in the ECG, ST segment is important to diagnose the ischemia. ST elevation occurs in the disease.

Diagnosis

The diagnosis is done on the basis of every 1-minute record and check how much time is taken to come back to normal. If 5 minutes is taken, then it is considered as serious coronary artery disease with symptoms such as dyspnea, chest pain, and decrease

in BP, ischemic ST, ventricular tachycardia, ectopic, and abnormal rise in BP.
1. **True positive:** Abnormal test in disease patient
2. **False positive:** Healthy patient shows positive
3. **True negative:** Healthy with normal
4. **False negative:** Patient having disease but test is negative

If the patient is sedentary, he/she can be tested using the tests like:
1. Thallium imaging
2. Coronary angiogram.

Treatment

- **Single block:** Balloon angioplasty
- **One or two blocks:** Stunt is done
- **Multiple blocks:** Coronary artery bypass surgery or grafting is done

ARRHYTHMIA AND SYNCOPE

Definition

The abnormal or irregular heartbeat is called arrhythmia.

Tachycardia: A heartbeat that is too fast is called tachycardia.

Bradycardia: A heartbeat that is too slow is called bradycardia.

Flutter or fibrillation: A heartbeat that is irregular in rhythm is called flutter.

Premature contraction: A heartbeat that is early than usual is called PMC.

Clinical features: For all the above conditions the following features are seen. They are breathlessness, dizziness and palpitation.

Interruption of electrical muscles leads to arrhythmia. The heart rate is 60–100 beats/min in resting position when person is fit and healthy.

Causes

Excess caffeine intake, hypertension, diabetes, hyperthyroidism, alcohol, smoking, stress, heart attack, congestive heart failure.

Diagnosis

EKG, echocardiogram, chest X-ray, blood, and urine test.

Risk Factors

Diabetes, hypertension, hyperthyroidism, hypothyroidism, old age, and heart problems.

Complications

Heart failure occurs by prolonged tachycardia or bradycardia.

Stroke: Stroke occurs when the blood supply to the brain is reduced or interrupted. It causes of supply of lack of oxygen and nutrients causes brain cell to die. Decrease of blood supply leads to formation of thrombosis and embolism in blood vessel also leading to the stroke.

Types of Arrhythmia

1. **Normotrophic arrhythmia:** The sinoatrial (SA) node is the pacemaker. This is divided into three categories. They are as follows:
   a. *Sinus tachycardia:* It increases the heartbeat. The clinical features would be syncope, dyspnea, dizziness, chest pain, weakness, and light headedness.
      Treatment:
      - *Medical:* Medication decreases episodes of tachycardia and helps in proper electrical conduction of heart.
      - *ICD:* Implantable cardioverter defibrillator. This monitors heart rhythm and stimulates the heart to return to normal rhythm.
      - *Coronary artery bypass surgery:* Grafting to coronary artery to increase blood supply to the heart muscle.
   b. *Sinus bradycardia:* Decreased heartbeat. The clinical features are confusion, dizziness, fatigue, shortness of breath, syncope, sweating, angina, and difficulty when exercising. Treatment is, if there is no cause diagnosed, then pacemaker is used. It is the device that uses electrical pulse to initiate the heart to beat at a regular HR. If there is a cause, then treatment can be given by medication.
   c. *Sinus arrhythmia:* This is an irregular pattern of breathing. Few patients have symptoms and few do not. The symptoms would be dizziness, syncope, palpitation, angina (chest pain), weakness, and dyspnea.
      Treatment: Based on the type of arrhythmia, they are atrial fibrillation and atrial flutter.
2. **Ectopic arrhythmia:** The pacemaker is other than SA node. This is divided into three categories. They are:

a. *Homotrophic:* The impulse arises from the conductive system.
b. *Heterotrophic:* The impulse arises apart from the conductive system.
c. *Heart block:* Arrhythmia occurs when the impulses generated by SA node are blocked while passing through the conductive system of the heart. This is divided into two categories. They are as follows:
   i. *SA block:* The impulses are not transmitted from SA node to AV node due to defective internodal fibers.
   ii. *AV block:* The impulses are not transmitted from atria to ventricles due to defective conductive system. This is divided into two categories. They are as follows:
      I. *Incomplete heart block:* This is again divided into four types. They are as follows:
         A. *First-degree block:* There will be delayed conduction because of the AV nodal delay.
         B. *Second-degree block:* There will be partial heart block because some impulses produced by SA node fail to reach the ventricles.
         C. *Wenckebach block:* The conduction of the impulses from atria to ventricles is gradually decreased for every beat and finally one ventricular beat is missed.
         D. *Bundle branch block:* This is either right or left bundle branch block.
      II. *Complete heart block or third-degree heart block:* Complete AV block or third-degree heart block is the condition where impulses produced by SA node do not reach the ventricles, so the ventricles beat in their own rhythm independent of atrial beat called idioventricular rhythm. These are two types.
         A. *AV nodal block*
         B. *Infranodal block*
         C. *Extrasystole:* This is divided into three categories:
            1. *Atrial extrasystole:* Extra P wave appears immediately after regular T wave.
            2. *Nodal extrasystole:* P wave merged with QRS complex.
            3. *Ventricular extrasystole:* Extra QRS complex follows the regular T wave.
         D. *Paroxysmal tachycardia:* This is divided into two categories.
            1. *Atrial paroxysmal tachycardia:* P wave inverted with normal QRST complex.

Physiology

2. *AV nodal paroxysmal tachycardia:* This is a temporary block of one part of conductive system.
1. **Circus movement:** In this the P wave is absent.
2. **Wolff–Parkinson–White syndrome:** This condition is present at birth, and there is an extra-electrical pathway between the heart's upper and lower chambers causing a rapid HR.
3. **Lown–Ganong–Levine syndrome:** This syndrome has short P-R interval with normal QRS complex and T wave.
4. **Ventricular paroxysmal tachycardia:** The condition has ischemic area is excited abnormally by a series of extrasystole. The ventricles contract 200/min.
5. **Others:**
   a. **Supraventricular tachycardia (SVT):** The HR is 160-200 bpm.
   SVT is of two types:
   i. *Atrial flutter:* The conduction rate of the AV node is about 230-240 impulses/min. The flutter leads to fibrillation and seen in one area of atria.
   ii. *Atrial fibrillation:* The conduction rate of the AV node is about 300-400 beats/min. It is seen in older aged patients.
   b. **Ventricular fibrillation:** The conduction rate of AV node is about 400-500 beats/min. This occurs with a heart attack.
   c. **Long QT syndrome:** It occurs either genetically or by medication causes fainting and life-threatening condition.

Ectopic beat: The beat originating from different site other than original site is called ectopic beat. The ectopic beat can cause irregular rhythm.

One of the causes are stress, caffeine and nicotine.

Ectopic beat is of two types:
a. Premature atrial contraction (PAC)
b. Premature ventricular contraction (PVC): The PVC is of two types: Couplet is two PVC and triplet is three PVC.

Sinus neat alteration: This is of two beats—bigeminy is every other beat is a PVC and trigeminy is every third beat is a PVC.

Supraventricular ectopy: The ectopic beat above the ventricles, i.e in atrial or junctional areas. This is of two types—paroxysmal atrial tachycardia where heart rate is 100 to 200 beats per minute and supraventricular tachycardia is where heart beat is 150-250 beats per minute.

Ventricular ectopy: Ectopic beat originating in the ventricle. The rhythm is irregular. This condition has premature ventricular contraction. The P wave is absent and wide QRS is present.

It is of following types:
- Single PVC
- Multifocal PVC
- R on T PVC
- Two PVC: Couplet
- Three PVC: Triplet

Ventricular tachycardia (VT): There will be 4 or more PVC seen. The VT is of two types. Sustained ventricular tachycardia (VT) and nonsustained ventricular tachycardia (NSVT).

Sustained VT: The heart rate is about 100 beats per second in 30 seconds and severely decrease of cardiac output is seen. Its an emergency situation. Immediate medical treatment is necessary.

Nonsustained VT: There are 3-5 PVC are seen called salvos. It leads to lethal arrhythmias. The first treatment is control of arrhythmia.

Ventricular fibrillation: It is the condition with inadequate electrical stimulation. Ineffective cardiac output. This is emergency situation. Activation of advanced cardiovascular life support (ACLS) is important with medication and electrical defibrillation to survive the patient. Then once patient is stable then they need AICD (automatic implantable cardiac defibrillator).

Physical therapy treatment for electrical conduction abnormalities:

S. No.	Causes	Physical therapy management
1.	Ectopic beat due to stress, caffeine and nicotine	The patients education to quit smoking. The patients on physical therapy program should avoid smoking two hours before and after exercising or can lead to ectopic beat
2.	Premature atrial contraction (PAC) is ectopic beat from atria causing irregular rhythm	Cardiac out put is not compromised. Physical therapy intervention is appropriate. Physical therapist must check the hemodynamic response like heart rate, blood pressure before, during and after therapy for safety of the patient
3.	Supraventricular tachycardia	The patient has high heart rate in between 150 to 250 beats per minute so to bring heart rate down. Techniques like cardiac massage is performed. This massage stimulates baroreceptors located in the carotid bodies of carotid artery. The parasympathetic nervous system is stimulated to decrease heart rate. The other techniques used are coughing and Valsalva maneuver or breath holding technique

Contd...

Contd...

S. No.	Causes	Physical therapy management
4.	Single PVC or unifocal PVC	This is a benign condition and patient can participate in physical therapy program
5.	PVC increase with activity	Stop physical therapy treatment and check for hemodynamic response and compromised cardiac output
6.	Multifocal PVC: PVC from different sites in ventricles	This is serious condition. Physical therapist must evaluate the patient before beginning or continue the physical therapy program
7.	R-on-T phenomenon	Patient who are on physical therapy program should be monitored closely as there are chances of dysrhythmia leading to ventricular tachycardia. It is an emergency situation
8.	Two PVC, Three PVC: In both conditions High ventricular irritability is seen with altered left ventricular function and ischemia	The medical treatment would be improvement of arrhythmia control and physical therapy treatment can be conservative and depends on hemodynamic response. Physical therapist must check the hemodynamic response like heart rate, blood pressure before, during and after therapy for safety of the patient
9.	Sustained VT	No physical therapy treatment is recommended secondary to emergency situation but physical therapist can help for stabilization of cardio-pulmonary resuscitation (CPR) and activating advanced life support (ALS)
10.	Nonsustained VT	Physical therapy treatment is contraindicated until the patient is stable

SYNCOPE AND ITS MANAGEMENT

Definition

Syncope is the sudden and temporary loss of consciousness due to inadequate cerebral flow, also called fainting/passing out.

Causes

Blood pressure becomes too low. The causes that trigger syncope are blood pooling in the legs, dehydration, heavy sweating, overheating, exhaustion, bradycardia, and tachycardia.

Types

1. **Emotional syncope:** This syncope occurs due to emotional fainting, decreased cardiac output, decreased cerebral flow,

suppression of myocardium, and severe vasodilatation caused by the parasympathetic division of the autonomic nervous system.
2. **Postural syncope:** This is due to prolonged standing causes pooling of blood in lower limbs.
3. **Micturition syncope:** This is due to low BP while standing or orthostatic hypotension causes micturition syncope.
4. **Neurocardiogenic syncope/neurally medicated syncope (NMS)/reflux, vasovagal/vasodepression syncope:** This type is seen in children and young adults.
   Clinical features: Fainting, lightheadedness, warmth, tunnel vision, or visual gray out. Nausea causes: Stress or pain. This is due to cardiac arrhythmia, decrease in cardiac output, bradycardia, and heart block.
   It happens with standing. Treatment: Put the resident in reclining position that helps to restore consciousness, restore blood flow, and end seizures.
   Situational syncope: This is the type of NMS syncope seen in men. The causes are swallowing, violent coughing, and laughing.
5. **Effort syncope:** This is due to stenosis of semilunar valves, increased cardiac output because of the exercise strain.
6. **Cough syncope:** This is due to increased intrathoracic pressure, decreased venous return. Cardiac output results in fainting.
7. **Carotid sinus syncope:** This is due to tight collar dress cause decrease in HR and vasodilatation.
8. **Cerebral syncope:** It is defined as loss of consciousness secondary to cerebral vasoconstriction.
   Causes: Hypotension, tachycardia, bradycardia.
   Risk factors: Sudden cardiac death.
   Diagnosis: Initial evaluation: Measuring heart rate, blood pressure, ECG, exercise stress test and Holter monitoring. If results are unclear then these two tests are performed for diagnosis transcranial Doppler ultrasonography and head up tilt test.
   Treatment: Defibrillators and cardiac pacing.

ELECTROCARDIOGRAPH

Definition

The ECG is the record or graphical presentation of electrical activities of the heart which occurs prior to the onset of mechanical activities. ECG is the test that measures the electrical activity of the heartbeat. It detects cardiac abnormalities such as rhythm disturbances, e.g., ventricular tachycardia and atrial fibrillation, coronary artery blood flow disorders such as myocardial infarction and myocardial ischemia, electrolyte disturbance such as hyperkalemia and hypokalemia.

ECG has three main components—P wave is depolarization of atria, QRS is depolarization of ventricles and T wave is repolarization of ventricles. There is depolarization and repolarization during each heartbeat. ECG has 12 leads and 10 electrodes that are placed on surface of chest and extremities but measured from 12 leads and recorded for 10 seconds. With each heartbeat, depolarization starts in SA node (pacemaker cells) go to atrium to AV node, bundle of His and Purkinje fibers to left ventricle.

Uses

Helps to know the rate and rhythm of heartbeat, heart chambers size and position are known, tells about damage to conduction system and muscle cells of heart, effect of drugs and function of pacemaker.

Pathology

Myocardial infarction is heart attack where patient clinical features would be chest pain, shortness of breath, fainting, murmurs, and seizures.

Cardiac arrhythmia: It has multiple conditions with different rate of heartbeat like tachycardia, bradycardia, irregular heartbeat called flutter. Main feature of arrhythmia is palpitation.
Treatment: Digoxin, the side effects of this drug are QT prolongation is seen on ECG and electrolyte abnormalities like hyperkalemia.

Electrical Changes during Muscle Contraction

The muscle contracts when stimulated by a nerve.

Resting Membrane Potential

The potential difference between inside and outside of the cell under resting conditions is known as resting membrane potential (RMP). In human muscle RMP is –90 mV.

Action Potential

When the muscle is stimulated, a series of changes occur in the membrane potential called action potential. This occurs as follows:

1. **Repolarization:** The altering of the muscle polarized state by interior as positive and exterior as negative.
2. **Depolarization:** The coming back to normal state of negative inside and positive outside.

Electrographic Grid

The ECG amplifies the electrical signals from the heart. This is recorded on strip of paper. The ECG paper consists of 1 mm size vertical and horizontal lines.

Time

The time duration is measured using the vertical lines. The lines are 5 mm thick and 1 mm thin. The time duration for thick lines is 0.02 seconds and thin lines is 0.04 seconds.

Amplitude

The amplitude is measured by using horizontal lines. There are thick lines of 5 mm and thin lines of 1 mm. The interval in between two thick lines is 0.5 MV and interval in between two thin lines is 0.1 MV.

Speed of the Paper

Normal recording is 25 mm/s. If the HR is very high, the speed of the paper is changed to 50 mm/s.

Waves, Intervals, and Segments of Normal Electrocardiograph

S. No.	Wave, segment, interval	From–to	Cause	Duration (s)	Amplitude (MV)	Applied anatomy
1.	P wave	First wave, positive wave, called atrial complex	Atrial depolarization	0.1	0.1–0.12	Tall and pointed P waves indicate right atrial enlargement
2.	QRS complex	Initial ventricular complex Q wave is small negative R wave is tall positive S is small negative	**Q:** Depolarization of the basal portion of IV septum **R:** Depolarization of the apical portion of the IV septum **S:** Depolarization of the	0.08–0.10	0.3	–

Contd...

Contd...

S. No.	Wave, segment, interval	From–to	Cause	Duration (s)	Amplitude (MV)	Applied anatomy
			basal portion near atrioventricular ring			
3.	T wave	Final ventricular complex	Repolarization of the ventricular musculature	0.2	0.3	Abnormal T wave indicates acute myocarditis, left ventricular hypertrophy and hyperkalemia
4.	U wave	Insignificant wave of ECG	Repolarization of the papillary muscle	–	–	U wave is visible when there is lower heart rate >65 bpm
5.	P–R interval	Onset of P wave to the onset of the Q wave	–	0.18 is the normal value; if >0.2 then value is called av nodal delay	–	Short PR interval causes severe cardiac arrhythmias
6.	QRS duration	Onset of Q wave to the end of S wave	–	0.08–0.10	–	Abnormal QRS is of two types Tall QRS: Abnormal pacemaker or hypertrophy of 1 or both the ventricles. Small QRS: Seen in patients with pleural effusion, obesity and hyperthyroidism.
7.	Q–T interval	Onset of Q wave to the end of T wave	–	0.4–0.42	–	Abnormal QT interval, i.e. if the value is greater than or equal to 0.5 seconds then health care

Contd...

Contd...

S. No.	Wave, segment, interval	From–to	Cause	Duration (s)	Amplitude (MV)	Applied anatomy
						provider should be notified immediately
8.	S–T segment	End of S wave to onset of T wave	This is isoelectric	0.08	–	ST segment depression indicates unstable coronary artery disease. Patient should be under the supervision of health care provider

Electrocardiograph Leads

The surface of the body is connected to the ECG machine by means of two electrodes called ECG leads.

Types

1. Bipolar leads
2. Unipolar leads

Bipolar Leads

The electrodes are active and taken from two limbs. These are called standard limb electrodes. Each lead has two electrodes. These are as follows:

Lead-I: This is connected to right arm and left arm. Right arm is connected to the negative terminals of the instrument and the left arm is connected to the positive terminal.

Lead-II: This is connected left arm and left leg. The left arm is connected to the negative terminal of the instrument and the left leg is connected to the positive terminal.

Lead-III: This is connected to the left arm and the left leg. The left arm is connected to the negative terminal of the instrument and the left leg is connected to the positive terminal.

Unipolar Leads

The active electrode is from one of the limbs. The indifferent electrode is obtained by connecting the other two limbs through a resistance.

Unipolar leads are of three types. These leads are called augmented limb leads. These leads are:
1. **avr:**
    a. Active electrode is from right arm.
    b. Indifferent electrode is from left arm and left leg.
2. **avl:**
    a. Active electrode is from left arm.
    b. Indifferent electrode is from right arm and left leg.
3. **avf:**
    a. Active electrode is from left leg (foot).
    b. Indifferent electrode is obtained by connecting the two upper limbs.

Unipolar Chest Leads

The indifferent electrode is obtained by connecting the three limbs—left arm, left leg, right arm through a resistance of 5,000 Ω. The active electrodes is placed at six points over the chest are called V1, V2, V3, V4, V5, and V6. All the leads are arranged over intercostal space.

V1: Near right sternal margin
V2: Near left sternal margin
V3: In between V2 and V4
V4: On the midclavicular line
V5: On the anterior axillary line
V6: On the midaxillary line

Cardiac Surgery: Closed Heart Conditions and their Physical Therapy Management

The cardiac conditions requiring closed heart surgery are:
1. **Acquired heart disease:** This has two categories:
    a. Mitral stenosis
    b. Aortic stenosis
2. **Congenital heart disease:** This has two categories:
    a. Patent ductus arteriosus
    b. Coarctation of aorta

ACQUIRED CONDITIONS

Mitral Stenosis

Definition

Mitral stenosis is the narrowing of the mitral valve opening which results in reduced blood flow through the mitral valve from the left atrium to the left ventricle.

Mitral stenosis is the narrowing of the mitral valve where blood from left atrium to left ventricle flow is decreased. Mitral stenosis is of two types—congenital and acquired. Congenital mitral stenosis is seen in infants. The acquired type of mitral stenosis is seen in adults. The severity of mitral stenosis is of two types—mild and severe. In mild type of mitral stenosis, there may not be any symptoms in Infants whereas in severe type of mitral stenosis the symptoms can be like shortness of breath, fainting and disability occurs in 7-9 years if the condition is not treated.

Causes

1. Rheumatic heart disease
2. Lutembacher's syndrome: The patient will have symptoms of acquired mitral stenosis and atrial septal defect
3. Atherosclerosis
4. Endomyocardial fibrosis
5. Hunter syndrome: The patient will have symptoms of both cardiomyopathy and mental retardation.

Pathology

The obstruction to the left ventricular inflow results in rise in pressure in the left atrium and pulmonary circulation. The pulmonary blood flow needs a pressure gradient of 10 mm Hg between pulmonary arteries and veins. To maintain the pressure gradient, the pressure will be above 20 mm Hg and vasoconstriction occurs. This affects the muscular arteries of the lower lobe, which shows medial hypertrophy. The normal mitral valve is 5 cm². The stenosis mitral valve is 1 cm². The pressure in the left atrium is about 6–12 mm Hg. In stenosis in order to maintain the adequate cardiac output the pressure in the left atrium is increased to 30 mm Hg or higher, so left atrial dilatation occur. The side effects of this causes pulmonary edema, pulmonary hypertension, right ventricular hypertrophy and right ventricular failure and tricuspid regurgitation.

Types of Mitral Stenosis

1. **Leaflet type:** The valves are stiff, rigid, and calcified.
2. **Commissural type:** The valves looks like fusion of commissures.
3. **Chordae type:** The valves looks like chordae and are thick.

Clinical Features of Mitral Stenosis

1. **Pulmonary hypertension:** Dyspnea, cough with frothy sputum, hemoptysis
2. **Right heart failure:** Weakness, fatigue, edema of feet
3. **Atrial fibrillation:** Embolism, blindness, hemiparesis
4. **Valvular lesions:** Mitral regurgitation, aortic regurgitation, and aortic stenosis

Complications of Mitral Stenosis

1. Pulmonary edema
2. Right ventricular hypertrophy and failure
3. Tricuspid incompetence
4. Atrial fibrillation
5. Infections such as subacute bacterial endocarditis, bronchopulmonary infections
6. Embolism: Cerebral (hemiplegia, aphasia), pulmonary, and renal hypertension
7. Enlarged left atrium

Diagnostic Tests

X-ray chest
1. Enlarged left atrium
2. Enlarged right ventricle
3. Enlarged pulmonary conus
4. Lungs changes such as pulmonary congestion, pulmonary edema, pulmonary infarction, pulmonary venous hypertrophy
5. Calcification of the mitral valve

ECG
1. **Early stage:** Normal
2. **Later stage:** P wave will be absent

Echocardiogram
This is a diagnostic test, which outlines the heart movements, pumping movements of heart, provides the pictures of heart chambers and valves, provides information about poor functioning of heart valves, weak heart muscles and blood clots in the heart.

Diagnosis of Mitral Stenosis

1. Loud first heart sound is heard
2. Heart murmurs are heard in mitral area
3. Right ventricle is enlarged causing backward displacement of left ventricle
4. Diastolic heart murmur.

Treatment

The treatment for the mitral stenosis will be either medical or surgical.

Medical treatment for mitral stenosis
In mild cases or in the cases where surgery is contraindicated, following are the treatment modalities that needs to be followed:
1. Bed rest
2. Salt-free diet
3. Diuretics such as furosemide increases urine production so decreases blood pressure in the lungs by decreasing the blood volume
4. Beta-blockers or calcium blockers: Slow abnormal heart rate that causes atrial fibrillation
5. Anticoagulants for preventing embolism, blood clot formation, and atrial fibrillation
   Treatment of complications: If drug therapy fails, then surgical treatment is suggested.

Surgical treatment for mitral stenosis

Heart surgery is done to separate the fused cups. The valves that are badly damaged needs artificial valve surgical replacement. The types of surgeries done are as follows:

1. **Valvotomy**
   a. *A closed valvotomy:* In this procedure, an instrument is inserted through ventricle, which is passed through the mitral valve and then it is dilated within it.
   b. *An open valvotomy:* In this procedure, the heart is opened and the cusps of the valve mobilized under direct vision.
2. **Balloon valvuloplasty**: Transcutaneous balloon dilatation of stenosed valves is now being done with good success rate. In this type of surgery, the valve is stretched open, a balloon on the catheter tip is passed through the vein and heart. Once the balloon reaches the valve, the balloon is inflated and balloon separates the valve cusps.

Cardiac surgery is contraindicated in older patients with severe valvular deformity.

Advantages
1. Avoids major surgery
2. The valves will be free of stenosis.

Aortic Stenosis

Definition

It is a condition where narrowing of the aortic valve occurs causing decreased blood flow from left ventricle to aorta. Stenosis also affect the pressure in left atrium. It is serious and most common problem. It restricts blood flow from left ventricle to aorta.

Causes

1. **Valvular stenosis:** Rheumatic fever, atherosclerosis, and congenital malformation
2. **Subvalvular stenosis:** Congenital
3. **Supravalvular stenosis**

Pathology

Patient feels weak and can faint due to left ventricle has to work harder to pump blood to aorta secondary to narrowing of the valve and muscular thickening of left ventricular wall. So less blood flow causes heart failure, left ventricular hypertrophy. Myocardial ischemia also occurs lead to arrhythmias and sudden death. When the patient with left ventricular hypertrophy exercises the patient will have symptoms like dyspnea, angina and syncope secondary to decreased blood flow in systemic circulation.

Symptoms

1. Angina/chest pain
2. Syncope/fainting
3. Exertional dyspnea
4. Fatigue
5. Pulmonary edema
6. Sudden death
7. Palpitation
8. Decrease in activity level
9. Murmurs

Symptoms in congenital conditions

1. Breathing problem
2. Fatigue of exertion
3. Poor feeding
4. Unable to gain weight

Signs

1. **Pallor:** Pale, grayish white
2. **Cerebral anemia:** Headache, faintness, giddiness, insomnia, irritability, and depression
3. Chest pain

Diagnosis

1. **Pulse:** Raises slowly and falls slowly
2. **Blood pressure:** Low systolic pressure
3. Systolic murmur
4. Second heart sound is soft and absent

Risk Factors

If the aortic stenosis is diagnosed after the age of 60 years the patient may not see any symptoms until 70 or 80 years and the calcium builds up in flaps. But if aortic stenosis is seen as congenital condition then calcium builds up, valves become narrow and stiff.

Investigations

X-ray chest
1. Normal in mild cases

2. Dilated ascending aorta
3. Aortic valve calcified
4. Left ventricular enlargement

ECG
1. ST-T changes occur
2. Arrhythmia occurs
3. Heart block or left bundle branch block is seen.

Echocardiogram
1. Thickened, calcified, and immobile aortic valve cusps
2. Left ventricular hypertrophy

Complications

1. Pulmonary edema
2. Right ventricular hypertrophy and failure
3. Tricuspid incompetence
4. Atrial fibrillation
5. Infections such as subacute bacterial endocarditis, bronchopulmonary infections
6. Embolism: Cerebral (hemiplegia, aphasia), pulmonary, and renal hypertension
7. Enlarged left atrium

Treatment

1. **Medical:** In mild aortic stenosis
   a. *Beta-blockers- for angina*
   b. Avoid strenuous exertion and competitive sports
   c. Rest
2. **Surgical:** In severe aortic stenosis
   a. Balloon dilatation of aortic valve gives temporary relief from obstruction
   b. Aortic valve replacement with a prosthetic or tissue valve

CONGENITAL CONDITIONS

Patent Ductus Arteriosus

Definition

The ductus arteriosus is an opening between two major blood vessels from heart called ductus arteriosus. If the ductus arteriosus remains open after birth then it is called patent ductus arteriosus. The ductus arteriosus is a vessel which connects the aorta with the pulmonary

artery during fetal life. Normally, it closes within few hours after birth. When it remains open, blood from the aorta flows through to the pulmonary artery resulting in two main effects:
1. Reduction of blood flow to the systemic circulation
2. Overfilling of the pulmonary circulation

Small PDA shows no symptoms and there is no need for any treatment.

Large PDA has poor oxygen blood flow to wrong direction, weak heart muscles, and heart failure.

Symptoms

The child will be prone to
1. Respiratory infections
2. Bacterial endocarditis
3. Dyspnea
4. Angina.

Signs

1. The child looks small or undersized
2. Heart failure if the duct is very large
3. Heavy apex beat
4. Mild diastolic mitral flow, murmur may be heard.

Clinical Features

If the shunt is small, then there is no any symptoms seen; but when the ductus is large, growth development may be retarded. No disability in infancy but cardiac failure with dyspnea may be the first symptom. The blood flow from aorta to pulmonary artery is 10–12 L/min.

The small PDA has no signs and symptoms until adulthood but large PDA causes heart failure after birth and symptoms such as easy tiring, breathlessness, rapid heart rate, poor eating and poor growth, sweating while eating, and not gaining weight.

Risk Factors

The higher risk groups are girls, babies born prematurely, babies born at high altitude like 10,000 ft. Before birth the ductus arteriosus connects left pulmonary artery to aorta. It closes at the time of birth. But if present even after birth called as patent ductus arteriosus. The PDA is commonly seen in Turner syndrome and genetic condition like incomplete X chromosome or 1 missing chromosome, so there are 45 chromosomes altogether.

Investigations

ECG
1. Normal in infancy
2. Left ventricular and left atrial hypertrophy
3. Pulmonary hypertension associated with right ventricular hypertrophy
4. Prolonged PR interval

X-ray
1. Left atrial and left ventricular hypertrophy
2. Calcified ductus

Echocardiogram
Demonstrates the patent ductus arteriosus.

Color Doppler
Suggests the direction of the blood flow.

Complications

1. Pulmonary hypertension
2. Infective endocarditis
3. Congestive cardiac failure

Contraindications for the Surgery

1. Transposition of great vessels
2. Tricuspid or pulmonary atresia
3. Infective endocarditis
4. Congestive cardiac failure

Treatment

Surgical treatment
The PDA should be closed either using medication if doesn't work then surgery is the option because PDA not closed for longer duration causes reverse effect of increased blood volume and to prevent complications. If smaller PDA no treatment is required and it closes by itself.

Coarctation of Aorta

Definition

Constriction/narrowing of the aorta is called the coarctation of the aorta. The function of the aorta is to deliver oxygenated blood via systemic circulation to whole body. When the aorta narrows the force on heart increases to deliver the blood to systemic circulation.

Types of Coarctation

1. Preductal or infantile
2. Postductal or adult or juxtaductal
3. Pseudocoarctation

Causes

The common site of the constriction is distal to the origin of the left subclavian artery and the constriction is in the upper region of the ductus. Coarctation of aorta increases load on the left ventricle, which causes increased blood pressure leading to left ventricle hypertrophy. The patient will have bicuspid aortic valve.

Sex

More common in males.

Symptoms

1. Usually no symptoms are seen.
2. Hypertension causes headache.
3. Intermittent claudication and coldness of feet occur.
4. Shoulder pain due to the dilated collaterals.

Signs

1. The upper part of the body may be well developed and the lower limbs are underdeveloped.
2. Left ventricular hypertrophy is seen.
3. Continuous murmur is heard.

Clinical Features

Babies after birth, difficulty in breathing, irritability, difficulty in feeding, and pale skin. If treatment is not given heart failure occurs leading to death.

In older adults and children, chest pain, high blood pressure, nose bleed, headache, leg cramps, cold feet, and muscle weakness.

Investigations

X-ray
Dock's sign: The rib's inferior margin is notched. It is seen in 3-8 ribs secondary to pulsation of dilated collateral arteries and collateral

blood flow occurs from subclavian artery to internal mammary artery to intercostal arteries.

ECG
1. **Infants:** The ECG will be normal.
2. **Adults:** The left ventricular hypertrophy and left atrial enlargement occurs.

Echocardiography and color Doppler
Echocardiography: This is a diagnostic test, which gives information regarding intracardiac anatomy and intracardiac anomalies.

Color Doppler: This is diagnostic test gives information about new observation and color flow diameter of evaluation.

Digital subtraction angiograph
This is a diagnostic test, which helps to clearly visualize blood vessels in bony and soft tissue structures.

Diagnosis

1. Left arm is underdeveloped
2. Left radial pulse is weak
3. Right side rib notching occurs.

Associated

1. Patent ductus arteriosus
2. Ventricular septal defect
3. Bicuspid aortic valve defect
4. Congenital aortic stenosis.

Complications

1. Infective endocarditis
2. Congestive cardiac failure
3. Hypertension and its complications
4. Subarachnoid hemorrhage
5. Aortic rupture
6. Premature coronary artery disease.

Treatment

Medical
1. Sedation
2. Antihypertensives
3. Prophylaxis for infective endocarditis
4. Treatment for left ventricular hypertrophy.

Surgical

Between 5 and 20 years of age:
1. Balloon angioplasty (dilatation of the coarctation)
2. Dacron or Teflon graft and end-to-end anastomosis
3. Aortic valve repair
4. Restrict energetic activities for 6 months postoperatively
5. Postsurgical hypertension is common
6. Follow-up for premature coronary artery disease.

PHYSICAL THERAPY MANAGEMENT FOR CLOSED HEART CONDITIONS

The resident is referred to physical therapy management. The physical therapy treatment is divided in to two types:

1. ***Physical therapy evaluation:***
   - First physical therapy evaluation is done
   - Submaximal test is performed to know the functional capacity of the patient. There are maximal and submaximal stress tests. The patients with cardiovascular conditions are tested using submaximal stress test secondary to decreased functional capacity and decreased tolerance to maximal test and also for the safety of the patient.
   - Based on the test aims and goals are planned and rehabilitation program is made. The physical therapy program is of two types—conservative physical therapy when the patient is on going medical treatment. If this fails and if patient requires surgical treatment. The physical therapy program is divided into two phases. Preoperative physical therapy program and postoperative physical therapy program.
   - The rehabilitation is called cardiopulmonary rehabilitation program where the focus on improving the functional capacity of cardiovascular system and pulmonary system so to return the resident to prior level of function.
2. ***Conservative physical therapy:*** The patient is on going medical treatment and along with that patient will participate in rehabilitation program.

S. No.	Aims of physical therapy	Plans of physical therapy
1.	To maintain range of motion	Active exercises
2.	To maintain the strength of muscles	Resistance exercises using Therabands and weights

Contd...

Contd...

S. No.	Aims of physical therapy	Plans of physical therapy
3.	To train the patient for vital sign monitoring	Heart rate, oxygen saturation, blood pressure monitoring and carrying pulse oximeter all times to know heart rate and oxygen saturation
4.	To train postural awareness	Postural education, ergonomic training
5.	To prevent venous pooling after aerobic exercise	Stretching is performed to muscles like hamstrings, quadriceps, upper limb muscles like biceps, triceps and scapular muscles
6.	To encourage warm up and cool down	Warm up is important for cardiac patient so maintain stable vital signs and prevent cardiac arrest
7.	To include balance training	Static and dynamic balance activities
8.	To include gait training	To focus on proper gait training, avoid abnormal gait and use of assistive devices if necessary
9.	To include stair climbing training	Ascending and descending stair climbing using siderails
10.	To train for energy conservation	Activity pacing and energy conservation, prevent fatigue

Surgical Physical Therapy Management

The physical therapy program for a patient who will be undergoing surgery is divided into two types and four phases:

Types

1. *Preoperative surgical physical therapy:* The preoperative training helps the patient mentally and physically ready for the surgery and also helps to prevent any complications.
2. *Postoperative physical therapy:* This training helps the patient to return to prior level of function.

Phases of Physical Therapy Program

1. Phase I or inpatient cardiac rehabilitation: In hospital, monitor vital signs, effects of bed rest, decrease risk factors.
2. Phase II—convalescent stage or recovery stage: Vital signs monitor, moderate exercise regime 6-8 weeks.
3. Phase III—maintenance stage: Risk factors modification, community exercise program.

Cardiac Surgery: Closed Heart Conditions and their Physical Therapy...

4. **Phase IV or commitment phase or ongoing for the life phase:** This phase includes diet, behavior modification, monitoring vital signs, home exercise program.

The following are the aims and goals:

S. No.	Aims of physical therapy	Plans of physical therapy
1.	To monitor the vital signs	The important vital signs to be monitored are heart rate, oxygen saturation and blood pressure
2.	To decrease the effects of bed rest	Frequent changing of positions in bed-like performing bed mobility, sitting with head end of the bed raised, sitting at the edge of the bed, chair at least few times as tolerated after surgery
3.	To decrease the risk factors	Ambulate short distances as tolerated
4.	To perform exercise program	Include warm up, aerobic exercises, cool down as tolerated
5.	Home exercise program	Walking, aerobic exercises, strengthening exercises to maintain good health and prevent complication, return to prior level of functions

Pulmonary rehabilitation program: This is a physical therapy intervention to train the pulmonary system effectively and efficiently to perform its functions. Patient is trained with the special techniques that helps to maintain and get back to shape.

S. No.	Aims of physical therapy	Plans of physical therapy
1.	To mobilization and removal of secretion	Active and passive techniques are used. Active technique where the patient performs by himself and passive techniques where physical therapist helps patient to perform the technique to remove secretions. Passive techniques are postural drainage, percussion, vibration and forced expiratory techniques like coughing and huffing *Active techniques:* ACBT (active cycle breathing techniques), thoracic expansion exercises, forced expiratory techniques like coughing and huffing
2.	To improve breathing efficiency	Breathing exercises like diaphragmatic breathing, segmental breathing, lateral costal breathing, glossopharyngeal breathing, and pulse lip breathing
3.	To teach postural awareness	Postural education and ergonomic training

Contd...

Contd...

S. No.	Aims of physical therapy	Plans of physical therapy
4.	To strengthen the muscles	Strengthening exercises using Theraband and weights
5.	To teach energy conservation and reduce fatigue	Activity pacing and energy conservation techniques
6.	To reduce stress	Yoga and medication
7.	To teach home exercise program	Warm up, aerobic exercises and cool down (stretching upper limb and lower limb muscles to prevent venous pooling)

The cardiac and pulmonary rehabilitation are the specially designed program for patients suffering from both cardiac and pulmonary conditions. The rehabilitation program helps the patient to return to their prior level of function.

Cardiac Surgery: Open Heart Surgery Conditions and their Physical Therapy Management

CHAPTER 4

1. **Congenital conditions:**
   a. Atrial septal defect (ASD)
   b. Ventricular septal defect (VSD)
   c. Pulmonary stenosis
   d. Tetralogy of Fallot (TOF)
   e. Transposition of great vessels
   f. Atrioventricular (AV) malformation
2. **Acquired conditions:**
   a. Mitral stenosis
   b. Mitral regurgitation
   c. Aortic stenosis
   d. Aortic regurgitation
   e. Coronary artery disease (CAD)

CONGENITAL CONDITIONS

Atrial Septal Defect

Definition

Atrial septal defect is the opening in the interatrial septum due to the deficiency in the septal tissue or hole in the wall called septum that divides both the atria of the heart. The smaller size hole closes by itself. If medium or bigger size hole needs a surgery. ASD is a congenital defect. It is the most common congenital heart defect. Small defects may close during infancy or early childhood on their own. Large defect can damage the lungs and the heart. Undetectable ASD lead to heart failure or high blood pressure (BP) (pulmonary hypertension).

Types

1. Fossa ovalis defect
2. Sinus venosus defect
3. Partial atrioventricular canal defect
4. Coronary sinus defects

Etiology

Congenital conditions are usually genetic cause because of chromosome abnormality, environmental exposure and defect in the genes causing heart conditions.

Signs and Symptoms

Children with moderate defects often do not develop any signs and symptoms until late teens. The chief signs and symptoms are as follows:
1. Failure to thrive
2. Tendency to develop chest infections
3. Untreated patients develop pulmonary hypertension in their late twenties to thirties.

Clinical Features

1. Dyspnea
2. Chest infections
3. Cardiac failure
4. Arrhythmias
5. Stroke
6. Fatigue
7. Shortness of breath
8. Heart murmurs
9. Heart palpitation
10. Swelling of abdomen, feet, and legs

Investigations

X-ray
1. Dilatation of the pulmonary arteries
2. Enlargement of the heart
3. Right ventricular and right atrial hypertrophy

ECG
1. Right ventricular hypertrophy
2. Right atrial hypertrophy
3. Right bundle branch block
4. Atrial fibrillation

Echocardiogram
It shows defects in the septum.

Diagnosis

1. Right ventricular hypertrophy
2. Wide fixed split of second heart sound
3. Systolic murmur on pulmonary ejection and mid-diastolic murmur on tricuspid flow
4. Pulmonary hypertension

Associated Lesions

1. Pulmonary stenosis
2. Mitral stenosis

Complications

1. Pulmonary hypertension
2. Infective endocarditis
3. Eisenmenger's complex (pulmonary hypertension)

Treatment

Surgical treatment

Surgery is done to repair ASD. Operative repair is the treatment for closure of ASD. It is done by implantable closure device by cardiopulmonary bypass.

Indications

1. Pulmonary to systemic blood flow >1.5:1
2. Pulmonary to systemic valvular resistance <0.7:1

Contraindications

1. Small defects
2. Pulmonary hypertension
3. Associated malformations
4. Coronary artery disease

Ventricular Septal Defect

Definition

The opening in the ventricular septum that causes contact between the two ventricles is called VSD. Ventricular septal defect is the hole in the heart which may be present at birth and is a congenital defect.

Pathology

The VSD is abnormal connection in between right ventricle and left ventricle. The blood passes between left ventricle to right ventricle.

Small VSD causes no problems and close on their own. Medium or large VSD need surgical repair to prevent complications.

Normally, right-side of the heart pumps deoxygenated blood to the lungs for oxygenation of the blood and left-side heart pumps oxygenated blood to the rest of the body. VSD causes the oxygenated blood from left ventricle is mixed with the deoxygenated blood from the right ventricle causing increasing load on the heart as mixed blood promotes less oxygen to the body tissues.

In fetus the ventricles are not fully developed. Genetic and environmental factors may play a role. VSD sizes are classified into three categories. They are small, medium and large. The small VSD is diameter less than or equal to 3 mm, the medium VSD diameter is 3 to 6 mm and large VSD diameter is greater than 6 mm. Acquired VSD can occur later in life secondary to heart attack or as complications of heart surgeries.

Sites

1. Membranous portion
2. Muscular portion
3. Infundibular portion

Causes

1. Pulmonary atresia
2. Tricuspid atresia
3. Transposition of the great vessels
4. Pulmonary stenosis
5. Patent ductus arteriosus
6. ASD
7. Coarctation of aorta
8. Mitral valve deformities such as mitral stenosis and mitral incompetence

Clinical Features

1. Pansystolic murmur is heard at the left sternal edge
2. A small defect produces a loud murmur
3. A large defect produces a soft murmur
4. Easy fatigue, poor eating, breathlessness, no weight gain

5. In adults, signs would be shortness of breath and heart murmurs
6. When the patient has symptoms like irregular heart beat, fatigue, shortness of breath when lying down or during exertion, the doctor should be notified immediately.

Investigations

The VSD heart defect is suspected if the murmur is heard. VSD is diagnosed in fetus using ultrasound scanning. The smaller the VSD defect, it is difficult to be noticed.

X-ray
1. Pulmonary plethora
2. Cardiomegaly (heart is enlarged)
3. Biventricular hypertrophy
4. Lungs have extra fluid

ECG
1. ECG shows heart defect or rhythm
2. Biventricular hypertrophy
3. Right bundle branch block

Echocardiogram with Doppler
It shows the VSD and other associated anomalies, helps to know the size, location, and severity. Also used during pregnancy called fetal echocardiogram to diagnose VSD.

Cardiac catheterization
1. Diagnose congenital heart disease
2. Function of heart valves and chambers

Pulse oximeter
Measures oxygen level in blood.

Associated Lesions

1. Aortic regurgitation
2. Complete heart block
3. Infective endocarditis
4. Eisenmenger's complex

Diagnosis

1. Recurrent respiratory infections of childhood, a failure to thrive
2. Moderately collapsing pulse
3. Biventricular hypertrophy
4. Pansystolic murmur

Complications

1. Complete heart block
2. Infective endocarditis on the right ventricular side
3. Pulmonary embolism
4. Lung abscess
5. Eisenmengers syndrome is seen in congenital conditions like ASD, VSD, PDA. The longstanding left to right cardiac shunt causes pulmonary hypertension. Pulmonary hypertension is a serious condition, it is high blood pressure in arteries of the lung. Arteries become hard and narrow and heart has to work harder to pump the blood to both pulmonary and systemic circulation.
6. Abnormal heart rhythm and valve problems

Risk Factors

VSD is seen in Down syndrome. It is a genetic condition. If the first child develops the heart defect, the parents should go for genetic counseling to know the risk or possibility of 2nd child getting the same. So parents have to plan accordingly.

Prevention

1. Early prenatal care
2. Genetic counseling if there is a family history
3. Diabetic management
4. Balanced diet (folic acid and limit caffeine) and regular exercise
5. Update vaccination before and during pregnancy
6. Avoid alcohol, drugs, and tobacco during pregnancy

Management

Around 30–50% close spontaneously if it is muscular or membranous.

Indication
1. Failure to thrive
2. Large defect <1 cm
3. Left-to-right shunt
4. Cardiomegaly
5. Right systolic pressure <65%
6. Pulmonary to systemic blood flow ratio is >1.5:1
7. Pulmonary to systemic vascular resistance is <0.5:1

Contraindication
Eisenmenger's syndrome.

Prognosis

Adults with closed VSD has good and normal lifespan. Patients with VSD if not treated die in Second or third decade. Lung transplantation is the treatment. But few of the patient can survive without treatment till fifth decade.

Surgical treatment

The surgical treatment can be lung transplantation, suturing a patch of dacron or pericardium to the VSD defect.

Pulmonary Stenosis

Definition

Pulmonary stenosis is the narrowing of the pulmonary valve resulting in diminished blood flow to the pulmonary circulation. This is a congenital condition in which obstruction of blood flow from RV to pulmonary artery occurs at one or more points leading to the decreased blood flow to the lung. In few patients, there is abnormal pulmonary valve formation called pulmonary atresia causing decreased blood flow to the lung.

Etiology

1. Congenital
2. Carcinoid syndrome
3. Associated with Fallot's tetralogy
4. The stenosis occurs above the pulmonary valve in the pulmonary artery. Right ventricle works harder to eject blood flow to pulmonary artery and so RV muscle thickens leading to hypertrophy.

Signs and Symptoms

1. Dyspnea
2. Cyanosis
3. Fatigue

Clinical Features

1. Loud harsh murmur
2. Right heart failure
3. Right ventricular hypertrophy
4. Right ventricular dilatation

Pathology

Pulmonary stenosis is of two types: Mild to moderate and critical. Mild to moderate can be detected. But the patient may not show any symptoms. The critical stenosis is seen in newborn babies. The main symptom can be cyanosis (Bluish coloration of skin lips and nail beds secondary to less oxygen in the blood).

Investigations

X-ray
Prominent pulmonary artery

ECG
In mild condition ECG is normal, and in moderate to severe condition ECG shows right atrium and right ventricle hypertrophy and enlargement of right ventricle.

Echocardiogram
This helps for diagnosis of pulmonary stenosis and seen as abnormal pulmonary valve thickening.

Cardiac catheterization
It shows degree of pulmonary stenosis, measures above and below the valve to know the amount of obstruction. Elevated right ventricular systolic pressure with low pressure in pulmonary artery.

Doppler study
It shows degree of obstruction.

Complications

1. Atrial fibrillation
2. Infective endocarditis

Treatment

For critical infants, immediate surgery is required with balloon dilatation of the valve.

The children with severe stenosis shows symptoms like fatigue and shortness of breath. This group requires open heart surgery. For children with critical stenosis balloon dilatation, pulmonary valvotomy, partial vulvectomy, transannular patch from right ventricle to pulmonary artery are done.

Tetralogy of Fallot

Definition

Tetralogy of Fallot is a condition in which four abnormalities occur. The dextroposition of aorta is aorta sitting in the middle of right ventricle and left ventricle but in normal situation aorta comes from left ventricle.

Etiology

This is a congenital condition in which there is an abnormal development of the bulbar septum which separates the ascending aorta from the pulmonary artery. This causes deoxygenated blood circulation in whole body hence causing cyanosis. It is diagnosed after birth or infancy. Pulmonary stenosis is narrowing of pulmonary artery. It is in between RV to pulmonary artery leading to lungs causing decreased blood flow to the lungs. Few have abnormal formation of pulmonary valve called pulmonary atresia causing decreased blood flow to lung.

Ventricular septal defect: It is the defect of septum between RV and left ventricle. Right ventricle takes deoxygenated blood to lungs, left ventricle takes oxygenated blood to whole body. In VSD the blood flow decreases causing decreased systemic circulation to the body which weakens the heart.

Over-riding of aorta: Normally left ventricle to aorta, the blood flows. In TOF aorta shifted to right and located above VSD. Aorta receives blood both from RV the deoxygenated, left ventricle is oxygenated. Right ventricular hypertrophy is condition where the heart muscles overwork leading to muscle thickening so heart becomes weak, stiff and fails to work. A few children may have ASD, coronary arterial abnormalities, and right aortic arch abnormality.

Clinical Features

- Cyanosis
- Fallot's spell
- Heart murmurs
- Fatigue
- Poor weight gain
- Irritability
- Clubbing of fingers and toes

- Shortness of breath
- Rapid breathing during exercise.

Fallot's spells or tet spells: It is rapid dropping of oxygen in the blood. These spells are seen in 2 to 4 month old. The spells cause due to apnea and lead to loss of consciousness. When toddlers and older kids have shortness of breath they squat as squatting increases lungs blood flow. Cyanosis is seen in the infants so if the baby is cyanotic (blue coloration) put baby into side-lying and pull the knees to the chest.

Signs
1. Clubbing of fingers or toes
2. Stunting of growth
3. Polycythemia

Symptoms
1. **Cyanosis:** It is bluish discoloration of the skin secondary to inadequate oxygen in the blood or poor circulation. It is of two types:
   i. Peripheral cyanosis: Seen in hands and feet.
   ii. Central cyanosis: Seen in lips and tongue. This central cyanosis occurs due to low oxygen in arterial blood secondary to lung or heart disorders.
2. **Syncope:** The syncope is due to the cerebral anoxia during the emotional upset.
3. **Squatting:** The child tends to adopt to a squatting position. This compresses the abdominal aorta and femoral arteries and raises the resistance in the systemic circulation which decreases the shunt of blood from right to left through the septal defect.
4. **Dyspnea on exertion:** On exertion, the oxygen content of the blood gets diminished in the systemic circulation.

Risk Factors

- Rubella infection during pregnancy
- Parents with TOF
- Down syndrome or DiGeorge syndrome
- Poor nutrition
- Mother's age >40

Complications

The following are the complications:
- Bacterial endocarditis (the lining of heart and heart valves are infected by bacteria

- Blood clots in brain can lead to stroke
- Abnormal heart rhythm
- Heart failure
- Death.

Investigations

X-ray
Dilatation of pulmonary arteries, boot-shaped heart secondary to RV enlargement.

ECG
Right ventricular hypertrophy, RA enlargement, and irregular heart rhythm.

Echocardiogram
Aorta is not continuous with AV septum.

Pulse oximeter
It measures oxygen levels.

Cardiac catheterization
This measures pressure and oxygen level in chamber of heart and blood vessels.

Diagnosis

Heart murmur is the abnormal sound caused by turbulent blood flow and cyanosis.

Treatment

The treatment is of three types:
1. **The palliative treatment:** The palliative treatment is done for infants who are few weeks older to children of 5 years. Blalock-Taussig operation that connects a subclavian artery to the pulmonary artery.
2. **Curative treatment:** This is for the age group of 5-10 years. The septal defect is repaired, the pulmonary stenosis is released.
3. **Surgery:**
   Intracardiac repair: Shunt is placed both in babies and older children.
   Complications of surgery are:
   - Sudden cardiac death
   - Coronary artery disease
   - Arrhythmias

- Ventricular septal defect
- Chronic pulmonary regurgitation.

To prevent infections preventive antibiotics are prescribed, patient should get a regular dental check-up, maintain good oral hygiene.

Prognosis

The prognosis is good. Following conditions need to be identified.
1. Pulmonary stenosis
2. Recurrence of the septal defect

Transposition of Great Vessels

Definition

Transposition of great vessels is a congenital heart defect involves great vessels such as SVC, IVC, pulmonary vein, aorta, pulmonary artery. The aorta and the pulmonary arteries are reversed so that the venous blood circulates throughout the body and oxygenated blood circulates throughout the lungs. The vessels are in abnormal position.

Types

Transposition of great vessels is divided into three major categories based on degree of involvement, number of vessels involved. They are:

1. **Dextro-transposition of great vessels:** This type is seen in the infants called cyanotic congenital heart disease. The infant has cyanosis and turns blue from lack of oxygen in the blood. There are two parallel circulatory systems, which are created different from the regular circulation. Right heart pumps deoxygenated blood to aorta. Left heart pumps oxygenated blood to lungs via pulmonary artery.
2. **Levo-transposition of great vessels:** This is acyanotic condition. Basically arteries are transposed. Systemic and pulmonary circulations are connected. The RV pumps at low pressure, but in this condition, the blood pumps at high pressure against systemic circulation.
3. **Simple TOGV:** The third type of transposition of great vessels is simple type where transposition of great vessels condition is seen without heart defects.
4. The fourth type of transposition of great vessels is complex type where transposition of great vessels condition is seen with heart defects.

Clinical Features

1. Congestive cardiac failure by 4–10 weeks of age
2. Increase in the left atrial pressure
3. Pulmonary venous hypertension
4. VSD
5. Pulmonary vascular obstructive disease
6. Cyanosis
7. Hypoxemia in the first week of life
8. Heart enlargement by 2 weeks

Risk Factors

Gestational diabetes during pregnancy.

Investigations

ECG
Biventricular hypertrophy.

Chest X-ray
Heart is enlarged and has egg-shaped and superior mediastinum looks string-shaped.

Treatment

- **Phase I:** No treatment is required for newborn babies but when babies are 6–12 weeks of age, balloon atrial septostomy is done via cardiac catheterization. Use of atrial septostomy improves blood flow to lungs, increases heart pumping efficiently and reduces right heart pressure. Angiocardiography is also done. It is X-ray examination of heart and blood vessels using radio-opaque fluid by intravenous injection
- **Phase II:** Convalescent stage or recovery stage—vital signs are monitored, moderate exercise regime given for 6–8 weeks.
- **Phase III:** Maintenance stage—risk factors modification, community exercise program.
- **Phase IV:** Commitment phase or ongoing for the life phase—this phase includes diet, behavior modification, monitoring vital signs, and home exercise program.

Arteriovenous Malformation

Definition

The malformation that occurs in the systemic or pulmonary circulation is called arteriovenous malformation. It is abnormal connection between arteries and veins seen in both brain or spine. It is seen at birth and can cause rupture leading to bleeding into brain and spinal cord and symptoms would be seizures and headache.

Types

1. Single
2. Multiple

Location

Brain, neck, limbs, thoracic wall, heart, and liver.

Clinical Features

1. Prominent pulsations on inspection of the neck
2. Hepatomegaly if liver site is affected
3. Intracranial bleeding
4. Epilepsy because of parietal lesion
5. Progressive neurological deficits cause hemiparesis
6. Headache
7. Seizures

Investigations

1. Echocardiogram: Heart failure with structurally normal heart
2. Angiograph
3. Cerebral or abdominal ultrasonography
4. MRI

Treatment

- Embolism or radiation therapy
- Medical treatment with medication for seizures and headache
- Closing off vessels with radiation or catheter

ACQUIRED CONDITIONS

Mitral Stenosis

Definition

Mitral stenosis is the narrowing of the mitral valve opening which results in the reduced blood flow through the mitral valve and backpressure into the chamber behind the valve.

Causes

1. Rheumatic heart disease
2. Lutembacher's syndrome (acquired mitral stenosis + ASD)
3. Atherosclerosis
4. Endomyocardial fibrosis
5. Hurters syndrome (cardiomyopathy, mental retardation)

Pathology

There is obstruction of left ventricular inflow at the level of mitral valve secondary to thickening of mitral valve leaflets and left atrial hypertrophy occurs. The pulmonary blood flow needs a pressure gradient of 10 mm Hg between pulmonary arteries and veins. To maintain the pressure gradient the pressure will be above 20 mm Hg and vasoconstriction occurs. This affects the muscular arteries of the lower lobe, which shows medial hypertrophy. The area of the mitral valve is 5 cm^2. In stenosis, it is reduced to 1 cm^2. The pressure in the left atrium is about 6–12 mm Hg. In stenosis, in order to maintain adequate cardiac output, the left atrial pressure increases to 30 mm Hg or higher, and the left atrial dilatation occurs that results in pulmonary edema, pulmonary hypertension, right ventricular hypertrophy, and failure and tricuspid regurgitation occur.

Types of Mitral Stenosis

1. **Leaflet type:** The valves are stiff, rigid, and calcified.
2. **Commissural type:** The valves looks like fusion of commissures.
3. **Chordae type:** The valves looks like chordae and are thick.

Clinical Features

1. **Pulmonary hypertension:** Dyspnea, cough with frothy sputum and hemoptysis
2. **Right heart failure:** Weakness, fatigue and edema of feet
3. **Atrial fibrillation:** Embolism, blindness, hemiparesis
4. **Valvular lesions:** Mitral regurgitation, aortic regurgitation, and aortic stenosis

Complications

1. Pulmonary edema
2. Right ventricular hypertrophy and failure
3. Tricuspid incompetence

4. Atrial fibrillation
5. Infections such as subacute bacterial endocarditis, bronchopulmonary infections
6. **Embolism:** Cerebral (hemiplegia, aphasia), pulmonary, and renal hypertension
7. Enlarged left atrium

Investigations

X-ray chest
1. Enlarged left atrium
2. Enlarged RV
3. Enlarged pulmonary conus
4. Lung changes such as pulmonary congestion, pulmonary edema, pulmonary infarction, and pulmonary venous hypertrophy
5. Calcification of the mitral valve

ECG
1. Early stage will be normal
2. Later stage: P wave will be absent

Echocardiogram
This is one of the most valuable investigations to diagnose and assess the severity of heart muscles.

Diagnosis
1. Loud first heart sound is heard
2. Murmur heart in the mitral area
3. Backward displacement of the left ventricle by the enlarged RV
4. Diastolic heart murmur

Treatment

The treatment will be either medical or surgical.

Medical treatment
In mild cases the conservative treatment can be done or in the cases where surgical treatment is contraindicated the following protocol can be followed:
1. Bedrest
2. Salt-free diet
3. Diuretics such as furosemide
4. Anticoagulants for embolism
5. Treatment of complications

Surgical treatment
1. **Valvotomy:**
   a. *A closed valvotomy:* In this procedure, an instrument is inserted through a ventricle, passed up through the mitral valve and then dilated within it.
   b. The valvotomy is performed to open the valve. It is done by cutting the valve by opening the sealed leaflets. It is an open surgery procedure and done for pulmonary stenosis and mitral stenosis.
2. **Balloon valvuloplasty:** Transcutaneous balloon dilatation of stenosed valves is being done with good success rate in cases of noncalcified, mobile mitral valve, pregnancy and when cardiac surgery is contraindicated in the older patients with severe valvular deformity.

Advantages
1. Avoids major surgery.
2. The restenosis of the valve can be done.

Mitral Regurgitation

Definition

The regurgitation or incompetence in the valve that does not fully close when the chamber receives blood through the valve causing the blood flow back to the chamber. The mitral valve regurgitation is the condition where mitral valve does not close tightly leading to backward flow to the heart.

This condition is subcategorized into three categories:
1. Aortic stenosis
2. Aortic regurgitation, and
3. Coronary artery disease (CAD)

Etiology

1. Rheumatic fever
2. Aortic valve disease
3. Ischemic heart disease
4. Cardiomyopathy
5. Myocarditis
6. Mitral valve prolapse
7. Infective endocarditis
8. Damage to papillary muscle

9. Endomyocardial fibrosis
10. Congenital
11. Myocardial infarction
12. Shortness of breath
13. Fatigue
14. Rapid fluttering heartbeat
15. Dizziness
16. Heart murmurs

Pathology

In normal condition when the left ventricle contracts the oxygenated blood goes into the aorta for systemic circulation. In mitral regurgitation some of the blood regurgitate back through partially opened value thereby reducing the amount of blood going into systemic circulation. Due to this the left atrium gets dilated, patient will have pulmonary edema, breathlessness, increased left atrial pressure.

Signs and Symptoms

1. Cyanosis
2. Dyspnea
3. Cough and hemoptysis
4. Edema in ankles, feet, and abdominal area

Investigations

X-ray
1. Enlarged left atrium, left ventricle
2. Pulmonary venous hypertension
3. Pulmonary edema

ECG
Left atrial and ventricular hypertrophy.

Echocardiogram
Dilated left atrial and left ventricle.

Doppler's effect
It detects regurgitation.

Cardiac catheterization
1. Dilated left atrium, left ventricle
2. Mitral regurgitation
3. Pulmonary hypertension
4. CAD

Diagnosis

1. Water hammer pulse is bounding and forceful pulse with rapid ascend and descend. This type of pulse is seen in pathological conditions.
2. Loud third heart sound
3. Systolic murmur
4. Pulmonary hypertension
5. First heart sound is weak.

Complications

1. Embolus formation occurs which enters aorta then coronary artery and leads to occlusion.
2. Carotid artery embolism causes obstruction of the cerebral circulation and leads to hemiplegia.

Treatment

Medical treatment
1. Diuretics
2. Vasodilators
3. Anticoagulants
4. Antibiotics
6. Diet management including low sodium diet
5. Regular review

Surgical treatment
Indication: Deterioration of left ventricular function.

Procedure: Mitral valve repair or replacement is done by cardiopulmonary bypass technique where the valve, papillary muscle and chordae tendineae are totally removed. A prosthetic valve called Starr-Edwards ball or disk valve of Bjork are used and sutured with the rim of the original valve.

Postoperative complications
Thromboembolism.

Treatment
Anticoagulant therapy.

Aortic Stenosis

Definition
Aortic stenosis is the narrowing of the opening of the aortic valve which results in reduced blood flow through the aortic valve and backpressure into the chamber behind the valve.

Causes

1. Valvular stenosis: Rheumatic fever, atherosclerosis and congenital malformation
2. Subvalvular stenosis: Congenital
3. Supravalvular stenosis

Pathology

Obstruction to the left ventricular outflow in aortic stenosis leads to left ventricular hypertrophy. Myocardial ischemia occurs without coronary artery lesions which may lead to arrhythmias and sudden death. The increase in cardiac output is not possible on practicing exercise due to the obstruction to the left ventricular outflow and symptoms such as dyspnea, angina, and syncope are aggravated.

Symptoms

1. Angina
2. Syncope
3. Exertional dyspnea
4. Fatigue
5. Pulmonary edema
6. Sudden death

Signs

1. **Pallor:** Pale, grayish white
2. **Cerebral anemia:** Headache, faintness, giddiness, insomnia, irritability, and depression
3. Chest pain

Diagnosis

1. **Pulse:** Raises slowly and falls slowly
2. **BP:** Low systolic pressure
3. Systolic murmur
4. Second heart sound is soft and absent

Investigations

X-ray chest
1. Normal in mild cases
2. Dilated ascending aorta
3. Aortic valve calcified
4. Left ventricular enlargement

ECG
1. ST-T changes occur
2. Arrhythmia occurs
3. Heart block or left bundle branch block is seen

Echocardiogram
1. Thickened, calcified, and immobile aortic valve cusps
2. Left ventricular hypertrophy

Complications
1. Pulmonary edema
2. Right ventricular hypertrophy and failure
3. Tricuspid incompetence
4. Atrial fibrillation
5. Infections such as subacute bacterial endocarditis, bronchopulmonary infections
6. **Embolism:** Cerebral (hemiplegia, aphasia), pulmonary, and renal hypertension
7. Enlarged left atrium

Treatment
Medical
1. Avoid strenuous exertion and competitive sports
2. Rest and beta-blockers—for angina

Surgical
1. Balloon dilatation of aortic valve gives temporary relief from obstruction.
2. Aortic valve replacement with a prosthetic or tissue valve should be one for everyone with aortic stenosis.

Aortic Regurgitation

Definition

The aortic regurgitation is the incompetence of the aortic valve which does not fully close when the chamber receives blood through the valve causing the backflow of the blood to the chamber. The heart is pumping harder causing heart failure.

Causes

1. Rheumatic fever
2. Syphilis
3. Infective endocarditis

4. Congenital disorders, e.g., bicuspid aortic valve
5. Connective tissue disorders, e.g., rheumatoid arthritis
6. Hypertension
7. Trauma

Pathology

The blood flows back through the valve into the left ventricle. Blood pressure falls because of the reduced volume. The left ventricle dilates leading to hypertrophy.

Signs and Symptoms

The symptoms are not seen until heart failure occurs. But patient may have shortness of breath, pain in chest, murmur, enlarged heart, and forceful pulse.
1. Pallor
2. Cerebral anoxia
3. Chest pain
4. Shortness of breath
5. Fainting

Complications

1. Pulmonary edema
2. Right ventricular hypertrophy and failure
3. Tricuspid incompetence
4. Atrial fibrillation
5. Infections such as subacute bacterial endocarditis, bronchopulmonary infections
6. Embolism: Cerebral (hemiplegia, aphasia), pulmonary, and renal hypertension
7. Enlarged left atrium

Investigations

X-ray
1. Cardiac dilatation
2. Left heart failure

ECG
1. Left ventricular hypertrophy
2. T wave inversion

Echocardiogram
Dilated left ventricle.

Doppler effect
Pressure gradient can be detected.

Diagnosis
1. Diastolic murmur
2. Left ventricular failure
3. Water hammer pulse

Management

Medical
1. Antihypertensive drugs
2. Vasodilators to prevent progressive left ventricular dilatation

Surgical
Aortic valve replacement or repair.

Indications
1. Cardiac failure
2. Cardiomegaly
3. Deterioration of the left ventricular function

Coronary Artery Disease or Ischemic Heart Disease

Definition
Coronary artery is the major blood vessel of the heart. When there is damage or disease to the coronary artery there is narrowing and limitation of the blood flow to the heart secondary to plaque formation. So there is insufficient coronary blood flow to the heart causing heart disease called ischemic heart disease. In this disease there is imbalance between myocardial oxygen demand and myocardial oxygen supply.

Sex
Males are more prone than females.

Age
Above 45 years are more vulnerable.

Site
The most common site is left coronary artery.

Etiology

1. Atherosclerosis
2. Coronary artery spasm
3. Embolism
4. AV malformation
5. Aortic stenosis
6. Aortic regurgitation
7. Mitral valve prolapse
8. Cardiomyopathy
9. Collagen disease
10. Syphilis
11. Anemia
12. Beri-beri disease

Signs and Symptoms

1. **Pain in the chest:** The symptoms can vary from no symptoms to chest pain to heart attack.
   a. *Angina pectoris:* Pain spreads across anterior chest wall radiates to arms due to lack of blood supply leading to accumulation of metabolites stimulates nerve ending of myocardium.
   b. *Myocardial infarction:* Pain is more severe and long-lasting.
2. **Dyspnea:** Breathlessness, pulmonary edema, anoxia of the tissue, shortness of breath.
3. **Alteration of skin color:**
   a. *Bluish:* The color is because of peripheral cyanosis decreases cardiac output.
   b. *Gray and white:* The color is because of poor arterial supply.
4. **Clamminess and sweating:** Palms and face because of sympathetic nervous system reaction, lightheadedness.
5. **Decreased BP:** This decreases cardiac output.
6. **Altered pulse:**
   a. *Tachycardia:* Heart rate (HR) is increased and faster HR.
   b. *Bradycardia:* HR is decreased.
   c. *Heart block:* 40 beats/min.
7. **Pyrexia:** The increase of temperature for 1 or 2 days after occlusion leading to infarction. This is due to necrosis of myocardium.
8. **Pericardial rub:** The inflammation of the pericardium causes a sound is heard through a stethoscope called pericardial rub.
9. **Edema:** Heart failure leads to excess tissue fluid cause edema in feet and ankles because of retention of sodium and water by the kidneys.

10. **Hemoptysis:** Coughing of the blood because of rupture of the pulmonary vessel.
11. **Cerebral symptoms:**
    a. *Cardiac syncope:* Reduction of blood supply to the brain causes loss of consciousness.
    b. *Cerebral anoxia:* Causes faintness, giddiness, depression, and irritability.
12. **Abdominal symptoms:** Nausea, indigestion, and constipation are caused due to venous congestion anoxia and lack of arterial supply to the abdominal organs.
13. **Altered blood gases:** Sluggish low of blood causes a decrease in exchange of gases in pulmonary circulation and increase in systemic circulation.
14. **Cardiac asthma:** This occurs at night. Patients will be suffocating, coughs, frothy, and pink sputum because of left ventricular failure produces pulmonary congestion leads to pulmonary edema.

Clinical Features

1. Angina
2. Acute myocardial infarction
3. Ischemic cardiomyopathy
4. Cardiac arrest
5. Sudden cardiac death
6. Silent ischemia

Pathology

Sudden occlusion: If a large embolus or a thrombus blocks the left coronary artery, the myocardium of the left ventricle cannot pump blood with an adequate force to maintain the systemic circulation. The inadequate blood supply to the brain and the vital centers in the brainstem lead to unconsciousness and death.

Gradual occlusion: The collateral circulation is established or the heart muscle may be hypertrophied.

Complications

1. **Disorders of the cardiac rhythm:** Disruption of the smooth transmission of contraction through atrial and ventricular muscles produce arrhythmias.
2. **Heart block:** Coronary arteries supply the interventricular septum. Infarction occurs at this site causes partial or complete

interruption of impulses. So the disruption of impulse transmission is called heart block. SA node is impaired so ventricles and atria function independently.
3. **Heart rupture:** The severe infarct replaces muscle by fibrous tissue and gets ruptured by pressure of the blood by 2 weeks called heart rupture.

Treatment

1. **Self-care:** Exercise, weight management, quit smoking, diet management
2. **Medication:** Beta-blockers, calcium channel blockers, blood thinners, statins
3. **Medical procedures:** Coronary angioplasty, coronary stent
4. **Surgery:** Coronary artery bypass surgery

Angina Pectoris

Angina pectoris is the chest pain that occurs due to decreased blood flow to the heart. Angina pectoris is one of the symptoms of CAD.

Clinical Features

1. Pain is clenched first in the chest, jaw and neck
2. Heaviness
3. Tightness
4. Squeezing
5. Pressure (all the above symptoms can be sudden or over time)
6. Lightheadedness
7. Sweating
8. Fatigue
9. Dizziness
10. Heartburn
11. Nausea
12. Shortness of breath

Types

1. **Stable angina:** The predisposing factors are physical effort, cold weather, smoking, emotional upset, high altitude, sexual intercourse, straining at stool, etc.
   Treatment: Rest, nitrates.
2. **Nocturnal angina:** This occurs in the middle of the night due to the left ventricular failure. The predisposing factors are dreams

that cause the release of the catecholamines, full bladder, and hypoglycemia.
3. **Unstable angina:** This is also called preinfarction angina. The predisposing factors are recent angina <60°, stable angina with severe symptoms, angina at rest, angina following myocardial infarction.
4. **Prinzmetal angina:** The causes for this are coronary spasm, smoking, platelet aggregation, and beta-blockers.
5. **Postinfarction angina:** This occurs after 2 days to 8 weeks of the myocardial infarction.

Treatment

1. Self-care, exercise, smoking cessation, diet management, and weight loss
2. **Medication:** Antihypertensive drugs, beta-blockers, calcium channel blockers, and blood thinners
3. **Medical:** Coronary stent, coronary angioplasty, cardiac catheterization, and revascularization
4. **Surgery:** Hybrid coronary revascularization, and coronary artery bypass grafting

Cardiac Failure

Acute Cardiac Failure

The sudden inability of the heart to maintain an adequate circulation is called acute cardiac failure.

Causes
1. Main artery occlusion
2. Decreased BP
3. Reduced peripheral resistance
4. Hemorrhage

Chronic Cardiac Failure

The left coronary artery disease causes diminished function of left ventricle, pulmonary circulation congestion, systemic circulation congestion leading to decreased nutrition to tissues, edema in lungs, feet and ankles leading to chronic cardiac failure.

Congestive Cardiac Failure

It is the condition where both the ventricles are failed leading to congestive cardiac failure. First there is left ventricular failure followed by right ventricular failure causing congestive cardiac failure. In chronic condition the heart does not pump blood leading heart failure.

Clinical Features

1. Rapid heartbeat
2. Fatigue
3. Shortness of breath during exercise, when lying down and at night
4. Swollen legs and feet
5. Dry cough
6. Loss of appetite
7. Dizziness
8. Bloating
9. Excess urination at night
10. Weight gain
11. Palpitations

Risk Factors

1. Hypertension
2. Cigarette smoking
3. High serum cholesterol
4. Obesity
5. Anxiety, stress
6. Heredity
7. Life style
8. Occupation
9. Lack of regular exercise
10. Diabetes mellitus

Diagnosis

1. **ECG:** ST-segment depression or elevation.
2. **Stress testing:** It is done on treadmill or bicycle ergometer. The workload increases till ECG change occurs with symptoms such as pain, fatigue, and dyspnea.
3. **Thallium stress test:** This test is done by injecting thallium, while the patient exercises. Thallium is picked up only by normal myocardium. Ischemic areas would appear as perfusion defects.
4. **Echocardiography and Doppler effect:** This will diagnose both left ventricular thrombus and mitral regurgitation.

5. **Coronary angiogram:** This will diagnose blockage of coronary arteries, its location, and severity.

Prevention
Reducing the risk factors such as smoking, weight, animal fat intake, egg consumption, and work-related stress, also the patient is advised to do regular and moderate exercises.

Management
Conservative management
1. **Self-care:** Exercise, weight loss, diet management (low sodium diet), quit smoking
2. Drugs such as analgesics (morphine), sedatives (pethidine), anticoagulants (hepa), defibrillating drugs (lignocaine), diuretics, vasodilators, antiarrhythmia, beta-blockers, antihypertension drugs, and ACE inhibitors
3. **Medical procedures:** Cardiac resynchronization therapy
4. **Device:** Implantable cardioverter defibrillator

Surgical treatment
Heart transplantation, coronary artery bypass surgery where saphenous vein is used as a graft and placing a pacemaker are the options.

CARDIAC REHABILITATION PROGRAM FOR ACQUIRED OPEN HEART CONDITIONS

The patient is then advised to undertake cardiac rehabilitation program to improve his/her cardiovascular health. The process of cardiac rehabilitation regimen are as follows:
1. **Evaluation of the patient for undergoing cardiac rehabilitation program:**
   - Initial medical assessment of the patient is done.
   - Submaximal testing is utilized to measure the cardiopulmonary functional capacity of the patient. Maximal and submaximal tests are performed to assess the cardiopulmonary fitness in the patient. Submaximal exercise tests are commonly administered as they are safer than the maximal tests.
   - The cardiac rehabilitation program is planned on the basis of aims and goals of the tests. The cardiac rehabilitation program is divided into two modes of therapy—conservative physical therapy and physical therapy for surgical patients. The conservative physical therapy is advised when the

patient is under medical treatment. Physical therapy for surgical patients are provided for both preoperative and postoperative patients.

– This therapeutic modality is also known as cardiopulmonary rehabilitation which aims to enhance the functional capacities of both cardiovascular and respiratory system to enable the patient to restore the optimum level of activity.

2. **Conservative physical therapy:** Patient undergoing medical treatment will also take part in the cardiac rehabilitation program.

S. No.	Aims of physical therapy	Plans of physical therapy
1.	To promote range of motion	Teaching of active exercises
2.	To strengthen the muscles	Resistance exercises using Therabands and weights
3.	To assess the patient's vital signs	Monitoring of heart rate, oxygen saturation, blood pressure and carrying pulse oximeter to assess heart rate and oxygen saturation
4.	To train for postural correction	Educating about posture correction and ergonomic training
5.	To prevent venous pooling caused after aerobic exercises	Stretching of muscles like hamstrings, quadriceps, upper limb muscles like biceps, triceps and scapular muscles prevents venous pooling after aerobic exercise
6.	To induce warming up and cooling down	Warming up is significant for cardiac patients so as to maintain stable vital signs and prevent cardiac arrest
7.	To promote sense of balance	Static and dynamic balance activities helps in the attainment of balance
8.	To provide gait training	Proper gait training by refraining from abnormal gait and using of assisted devices
9.	To train for stair climbing	Exercises like ascending and descending stair climbing by the use of siderails
10.	To instruct for energy conservation	Activity pacing and energy conservation prevents fatigue

3. **Cardiac rehabilitation for surgical patients:** The physical therapy program for patients who will be undergoing surgery are discussed below:
   Types
   a. *Physical therapy for preoperative surgical patients:* This involves the conduction of exercises to strengthen the patient physically to avoid complications after surgery.

Cardiac Surgery: Open Heart Surgery Conditions and their Physical Therapy... 121

b. *Physical therapy for postoperative surgical patients:* This includes the training of the patients to rehabilitate their level of functioning.

Phases of cardiac rehabilitation program for surgical patients

1. *Phase I or inpatient cardiac rehabilitation:* This includes the hospital care focusing mainly on vital signs monitoring, observing the effects of bed rest and reducing the associated risk factors.
2. *Phase II or outpatient cardiac rehabilitation:* This stage includes the provision of care immediately after the hospitalization involving monitoring of vital signs and moderate exercise regime for 6-8 weeks
3. *Phase III or late recovery stage:* This involves the modification of risk factors and community exercise regime.
4. *Phase IV or maintenance phase:* This phase comprises of diet and behavior modifications, observation of vital signs and home exercises regime.

Aims and goals of cardiac rehabilitation program for surgical patients are discussed below:

S. No.	Aims of physical therapy	Plans of physical therapy
1.	To assess vital signs	Assessment of heart rate, oxygen saturation and blood pressure are significant to be measured
2.	To minimize the ill effects of prolong bed rest	Changing of positions in bed at every regular interval such as performing bed mobility, sitting with the raised head end of the bed, sitting at the edge of the bed or chair for few minutes as tolerated after the surgery could be of more help in decreasing the effects of prolong bed rest
3.	To reduce the associated risk factors	Ambulating patients for short distances as per their tolerance after the surgery
4.	To enable patients to perform exercises	Including exercises such as warm up, cool down and aerobic exercises as tolerated
5.	Home exercise program regime	Exercises such as strengthening exercises, walking, aerobic exercises are essential to promote sound health, prevent further complications after surgery and restore the prior level of functioning of the patient

4. **Pulmonary rehabilitation program:** Pulmonary rehabilitation is one of the treatment modality of physical therapy wherein the patients with respiratory disorders are trained for exercises

and breathing techniques to improve the lung capacity and its functions to rehabilitate their prior level of functioning.

S. No.	Aims of physical therapy	Plans of physical therapy
1.	To assist in the mobilization and removal of secretions	Teaching of active and passive exercise techniques. Active techniques are those exercises regime where the patient does the exercises by himself whereas passive techniques involves the physical therapist who assists the patient to remove the respiratory secretions. Techniques such as postural drainage, percussion, vibration and forced expiratory methods such as coughing and huffing are passive exercise techniques *Active techniques:* ACBT (active cycle breathing techniques), thoracic expansion exercises, forced expiratory techniques like coughing and huffing are the techniques of active passive exercises
2.	To enhance the breathing pattern	Breathing exercises such as diaphragmatic breathing, segmental breathing, lateral costal breathing, glossopharyngeal breathing and pulse lip breathing promotes better breathing efficiency
3.	To teach posture correction exercises	Education on postural correction and ergonomic training
4.	To improve the muscle strength	Strengthening of the muscles by the use of Theraband and weights
5.	To educate about energy conservation and ways to reduce fatigue	Technique like activity pacing can help in the energy conservation
6.	To calm the mind	Yoga and meditation
7.	To educate home exercises	Teaching of warm up, aerobic exercises, cool down (stretching upper limb and lower limb muscles to prevent venous pooling)

Both the cardiac and pulmonary rehabilitation programs are structured for patients with cardiac and pulmonary disorders. These rehabilitation programs assists the patient to get back to their optimal functioning capacity.

Thoracic Surgery 5

FRACTURE RIBS

Definition
The break in continuity of the rib bone is called fracture ribs. It is an injury when rib cage bone cracks.

Causes
Direct violence, accident, fall, and sports such as golf and prolonged coughing.

Clinical Features
1. Pain while deep breathing
2. Cough
3. Pain with twisting the body or bending the body
4. Pain with palpation or tenderness
5. Shortness of breath
6. Gritting sensation over injured area
7. Bruising
8. Inhibit deep breathing

Complications
1. Chronic bronchitis
2. Associated injury, e.g., kidney and spleen with lower rib fracture
3. Pneumothorax
4. Hemothorax
5. Damage to air passage
6. Pneumonia

Diagnosis
Radiograph: This shows the level of the fracture.

Treatment
Self-care: Ice packs.

Medical

- Analgesics for the pain relief for intercostal nerve block.
- Non-steroidal anti-inflammatory drugs (NSAIDs) to decrease fever, inflammation, and pain.

Physiotherapy

Breathing exercises are taught to the patient.

Physical Therapy Management

The patient is evaluated first. Then the intervention is planned with aims and goals according to the patient current health condition. The following is the generalized program:

S. No.	Aims of physical therapy	Plan of physical therapy
1.	To expand chest cavity	Stretching to shoulder and trunk muscles
2.	To improve breathing efficiency	Breathing exercises like diaphragmatic breathing
3.	To increase postural awareness	Postural reeducation, ergonomic set up at home and work
4.	To teach energy conservation, reduce fatigue	Activity pacing, paced breathing
5.	To improve range of motion	Range of motion exercises to all joints of upper limb, lower limb and trunk
6.	To teach strengthening exercises	Strengthening exercise to upper limb, lower limb and trunk using weights or Theraband

FLAIL CHEST

Definition

Flail chest involves multiple rib fractures broken anteriorly and posteriorly that makes the segment of the chest wall float. This is a life-threatening condition that occurs due to trauma. In this condition, at least two adjacent ribs are broken into two pieces.

Causes

- **Children:** Blunt force and osteogenesis imperfecta.
- **Adults:** Fall.

Clinical Features

1. Involved segment of the chest wall will be floating.

2. Segment is sucked in during inspiration and driven out during expiration, so breathing is called paradoxical breathing. The flail segment moves in opposite direction with the rest of the chest wall. For example, when the chest moves out the flail segment moves in and when the chest moves in the flail segment moves out called paradoxical breathing. This type of breathing is painful and breathing work effort is increased.
3. One side of the heart will be moving in while the other side moves out.
4. Shortness of breath.
5. Chest pain.

Signs and Symptoms

1. Hypoxia
2. Restriction in breathing
3. Severe pain
4. **Paradoxical respiration:** The sucked in segment during inspiration compresses the homolateral lung and drives out the air from it into the contralateral lung. This reverses during expiration called paradoxical respiration and results in high degree of carbon-dioxide retention. This causes stiffness in lungs as it requires extra breathing efforts and increases the lung resistance.
5. **Pulmonary contusion:** It is the lung bruise that causes blood oxygenation interference causing respiratory problem.

Treatment

1. Immediate hospitalization of these patients.
2. Relaxant drug is administered.
3. Endotracheal tube is introduced.
4. Intrapleural drains are given.
5. Positive pressure respiration is started.
6. Bronchial toilet may be required through bronchoscopy.
7. 10–14 days are required for union of fractured ribs.
8. Tracheostomy is performed. This is internal pneumatic fixation and is capable of managing many patients with this injury.
9. Patient should be under prolonged period of mechanical ventilation and longer stay in ICU is advised.
10. Old technique of operative fixation is preferred.

11. A long curved incision is made over the affected side and the pleural pace is entered by stripping the upper border of one of the ribs.
12. The bleeding from intercostal or internal mammary artery should be secured.
13. The flail segment are stabilized by inserting Kirchners wires or short rush nails through the medullary cavities of the ribs. Additional fixation by stout sutures through the intercostal muscles. Finally, thoracotomy is closed with tube drainage of the pleural cavity.

If untreated, sharp broken edges of the ribs can puncture pleural sac and lungs causing pneumothorax with paradoxical breathing and mediastinum shifts called mediastinal flutter. Flail chest and pulmonary contusion leads to respiratory failure.

Medication

- Intercostal blocks
- Opioids increases ventilation, tidal volume, and blood oxygenation.

Physical Therapy Management

Same as of Fracture (Refer page 124).

Chest physical therapy (PT): The chest physical therapy includes postural drainage, breathing exercises, coughing techniques, range of motion exercises, resistance exercises for trunk, lower extremities. For postural drainage the key for successful drainage is proper positioning according to the lobe for secretion removal. Range of motion exercises to prevent atrophy of muscles. Resistance exercises to upper extremity and lower extremity using weights and Theraband. Trunk exercises in sitting and standing.

All exercises should be performed three sets with 6-8 repetitions with rest in between walking.

Postural correction; before discharging the patient, teaching mobility exercises to core muscles for good positioning, mobility of chest, and pectoral muscle stretching.

STOVE IN CHEST

Definition

This is a rare condition in which multiple injuries occurs to the ribs. The segment of chest wall collapse leading to immediate mortality.

Clinical Features

1. Broken ribs
2. Cardiac injury
3. Pulmonary injury
4. Blood vessels damage

Cause

Car accident.

Complications

1. Contusion
2. Laceration of lung
3. Penetration of the pleural cavity
4. Injury to the air passage increases

Diagnosis

1. Repeated radiographs
2. Blood gas analysis.

PNEUMOTHORAX

Definition

The air present in the pleural cavity is called pneumothorax or the leaking of air into the space between the chest wall and lung.

Causes

Lung laceration due to fracture rib, blunt chest injury, lung disease, during a medical procedure, bullet wounds, hard hit with football tackle to chest, broken ribs, road traffic accidents.

Clinical Features

1. The air escapes from the bronchopulmonary tree into the pleural cavity.
2. The air in the pleural cavity will compress on the lung and produce difficulty in proper aeration.
3. Pain in the chest, coughing, low oxygen in the body, tachycardia, tachypnea, shortness of breath, shallow breathing.

Complications

If it is spontaneous pneumothorax and if small amount of air is trapped then no treatment is required as it heals by itself and no complications occur but if large amount of air is trapped then immediate intervention is required or may be fatal. Some complications of pneumothorax are—cardiac arrest, hypoxemic respiratory failure, pulmonary edema, hemopneumothorax, empyema, bronchopulmonary fistula.

Types

1. Closed pneumothorax
2. Open pneumothorax or traumatic pneumothorax
3. Tension pneumothorax
4. Spontaneous pneumothorax
5. Chronic pneumothorax

Closed Pneumothorax

The condition where the air comes out of the lung to enter the pleural cavity and no more air enters as the lung tissue is closed is called closed pneumothorax.

Causes
Contusion of the lung by fractured ribs.

Clinical features
Closed pneumothorax is absorbed and lungs re-expand. The time required for normal resorption depends on size of the pneumothorax.

Treatment
1. Air evacuated from the pleural cavity by direct aspiration
2. Pushing an intercostal tube through the second intercostal space anteriorly.

Open Pneumothorax or Traumatic Pneumothorax

Definition
This is the condition where air enters into the pleural cavity through a penetrating wound in the chest wall. Tension occurs if air around lungs increases in pressure. It is the cause of trauma and need immediate treatment.

Clinical features
The negative pressure in the pleural cavity will draw more air from outside, which will prevent proper aeration of the lung. The severity of the condition depends on the how big is the size of the opening. If the opening is bigger than size of trachea then leads to complete lung collapse because the air is entering through the wounds instead of entering through the trachea.

Diagnosis
The diagnosis of pneumothorax is done by using radiographs, CT scan, ultrasound imaging.

Treatment
Closure of the wound in the chest wall.

Procedure
This is done by a piece of gauze covered with elastoplast or with one or two skin stitches. Later, proper exploration of the wound and debridement should be carried out. Thoracotomy incision through the wound of the chest wall is done if required.

Tension Pneumothorax

Definition
The tension pneumothorax occurs when the air is trapped in the pleural cavity compromising cardiopulmonary function.

Clinical features
Air enters the pleural cavity during inspiration and exit is prevented during expiration. So, the volume of air is increased gradually in the pleural cavity that cause collapse of the lungs and a shift of the mediastinum to the opposite side.

Treatment
Immediate intervention as the condition is fatal. A wide bore needle is inserted through the second intercostal space of the pleural cavity, one and half-inches lateral to the sternum to avoid injury to the internal mammary artery. It is later replaced by water-seal drainage. If leakage present after 5 days thoracotomy is done.

Spontaneous Pneumothorax or Nontraumatic Pneumothorax

Definition
Spontaneous pneumothorax or non-traumatic pneumothorax occurs without any cause and it is the collection of air in the spaces located around the lung.

Causes
1. Congenital
2. Emphysematous
3. Tuberculous
4. Heavy weight lifting
5. Muscular strain

Onset
Sudden.

Clinical features
1. Chest pain
2. Sensation of compression

Types
Primary: This type is seen in young patients with no lungs problem.

Secondary: This type is seen in older patients with lungs problem such as COPD conditions like chronic bronchitis and emphysema, tuberculosis (TB), lung cancer, pneumonia, asthma, and cystic fibrosis.

Treatment
Mild cases: Pneumothorax is gradually absorbed. If pneumothorax persists, an intercostal tube may be inserted to remove the excess air and supportive treatment such as oxygen therapy is given.

Surgical treatment
Indication
Three or four recurrent attacks of pneumothorax on the same side.

If the other lung has already been involved, the surgery is urgently advised in order to avoid occurrence of bilateral pneumothorax.

Procedure
The type of surgery performed is posterolateral thoracotomy. The bleeding is controlled by hot packs. The lung is properly inspected to determine the site of air leakage. A large cyst should be unroofed and sutured. The chest wall is closed with underwater seal drainage.

Chronic Pneumothorax

This is also called persistent or recurrence of pneumothorax.

Treatment
A thoracotomy is performed and partial pleurectomy is done so that the visceral pleura will adhere to the chest wall obliterating the pleural space. If bronchopleural fistula is noticed, it should be sutured. The thoracotomy wound is closed with underwater seal drainage.

Surgical Physical Therapy Management

The physical therapy program for a patient who will be undergoing surgery is divided in to two types and four phases:

Types

1. *Preoperative surgical physical therapy:* This is training the patient to get ready and getting physically fit to prevent complications of surgery unless it is an emergency situation.
2. *Postoperative physical therapy:* This is training the patient to return to prior level of function.

Phases of Physical Therapy Program

1. Phase I or inpatient cardiac rehabilitation: In hospital, monitor vital signs, effects of bed rest, decrease risk factors.
2. Phase II—convalescent stage or recovery stage: Vital signs monitor, moderate exercise regime 6-8 weeks.
3. Phase III—maintenance stage: Risk factors modification, community exercise program.
4. Phase IV or commitment phase or ongoing for the life phase: This phase includes diet, behavior modification, monitoring vital signs, home exercise program.

The following are the aims and goals:

S. No.	Aims of physical therapy	Plans of physical therapy
1.	To monitor the vital signs	Heart rate, oxygen saturation using pulse oximeter. It is handy. Patient can carry easily and blood pressure
2.	To decrease the effects of bed rest	Frequent changing of positions in bed-like performing bed mobility, sitting with head end of the bed raised, sitting at the edge of the bed, chair atleast few times as tolerated after surgery
3.	To decrease the risk factors	Ambulate short distances as tolerated
4.	To perform exercise program	Include warm up, aerobic exercises, cool down as tolerated
5.	Home exercise program	Walking, aerobic exercises, strengthening exercises to maintain good health and prevent complication, return to prior level of functions

Pulmonary rehabilitation program: This is a physical therapy intervention to train the pulmonary system effectively and efficiently to perform its functions. Patient is trained with the special techniques that helps to maintain and get back to shape.

S. No.	Aims of physical therapy	Plans of physical therapy
1.	To mobilization and removal of secretion	Active and passive techniques are used. Active technique where the patient performs by himself and passive techniques where physical therapist helps patient to perform the technique to remove secretions. Passive techniques are postural drainage, percussion, vibration and forced expiratory techniques like coughing and huffing *Active techniques:* ACBT (active cycle breathing techniques), thoracic expansion exercises, forced expiratory techniques like coughing and huffing
2.	To improve breathing efficiency	Breathing exercises like diaphragmatic breathing, segmental breathing, lateral costal breathing, glossopharyngeal breathing, and pulse lip breathing
3.	To teach postural awareness	Postural education and ergonomic training
4.	To strengthen the muscles	Strengthening exercises using Theraband and weights
5.	To teach energy conservation and reduce fatigue	Activity pacing and energy conservation techniques
6.	To reduce stress	Yoga and medication
7.	To teach home exercise program	Warm up, aerobic exercises and cool down (stretching upper limb and lower limb muscles to prevent venous pooling)

HEMOTHORAX

Definition

Accumulation of blood in the pleural space is called hemothorax or collection of blood in pleural cavity, lungs or the chest wall.

Causes

1. **Chest trauma:** The sources of bleeding are from intercostal vessels, internal thoracic vessels, lung parenchyma, bronchial arteries, major pulmonary vessels, heart, great vessels.
2. **Blunt injury:** Also called penetrating injury which is associated with rib fractures.
3. **Iatrogenic:** Means treatment induced complications, e.g., chemotherapy treatment and side effects like wise postoperative thoracotomy surgery may cause injury to inferior pulmonary vessel, chest wall adhesions, bronchial vessels or intercostal vessels and other techniques are needle lung biopsy and core biopsy technique.

4. **Spontaneous pneumothorax:** Occurs when there is tear of vascular adhesion.
5. Pulmonary embolism
6. Tuberculosis.
7. **Neoplasm:** Lungs carcinoma with pleural or chest-wall invasion, metastatic lung or pleural disease, mesothelioma.

Clinical Features

1. Anxiety
2. Difficulty breathing
3. Low blood pressure
4. Rapid heart rate
5. Cold skin
6. Chest pain with breathing

Diagnosis

This depends on the type, location, and extent of the injury need to be considered. Physical signs suggest pleural fluid, confirmation is done by X-rays, upright and lateral view, and thoracentesis.

Management

General

Airway is maintained, placement of appropriate monitoring lines, IV access. Blood should be sent for group and cross match, hematocrit analysis, and associated injury.

Specific

Placement of chest tube at the 5th or 6th intercostal space.

Thoracotomy is required if the initial chest tube output is >1,500 mL, blood with hypotension, ongoing chest tube output is >300 mL/h or 3 hours.

If drainage is inadequate, thoracotomy is required to manage associated intrathoracic injuries or pathology.

Antibiotics helps to decrease infection.

Fibrinolytic Therapy: Helps in breaking down the clotted blood in pleural space.

Complications

1. Empyema
2. Fibrothorax with trapped lung

Treatment

1. Thoracotomy and drainage using chest tube
2. If fibrothorax is seen as there are chances of fibrosis and scarring leading to fusion of the layers and decreased pleural space around the lungs which leads to decreased movement of rib cage and lungs. If this happens then the treatment is called decortication. Decortication is a surgical treatment where removal of fibrotic tissue around the lungs is done so the lungs can expand. This technique is indicated for pleural cavity fibrosis and pleural cavity infection.

Physical Therapy Management

Same as of Fracture (Refer page 124).

HEMOPNEUMOTHORAX

Definition

The presence of blood and air within the pleural cavity is called hemopneumothorax. This is a complication of the thoracic injuries. Presence of air in the chest cavity is pneumothorax and blood in the chest cavity is called hemothorax. When the combination of both air and blood occurs secondary to injury to the chest or lungs is called hemopneumothorax.

Pathology

The chest wall and pleural space gets punctured. The air and blood enters the space and equalizes the pressure of atmosphere. So the two membranes of pleura does not adhere to each other. The rib cage moves out and does not pull the lungs so cannot expand the lungs. Pressure does not drop and no air can reach bronchi. Respiration does not occur leading to collapsed lung.

Clinical Features

1. Breathing problems
2. **Infection:** If not treated or removed a deposition of organized, fibrin will prevent proper expansion of the lung. The bleeding occurs because of laceration of the lung, surface, or damage to the intercostal artery or rupture of an intrapleural adhesion.

Complications

Pneumothorax.

Treatment

Tube Thoracotomy

It is the chest drainage. It drains between the ribs and into intercostal space. It removes blood and air so creates negative pressure, hence lungs functions normally. In order to close the insertion the surgery is performed. Transfusion to restore blood volume, aspiration of blood from the pleural cavity requires sedation of the patient. Tube drainage is indicated at 7th or 8th intercostal space on the midaxillary line, second tube is inserted at 2nd intercostal space. Both connected to an underwater seal drainage, if patient does not respond to this treatment thoracotomy should be carried out.

Physical Therapy Management

Same as of Fracture (Refer page 124).

Indications

When the bleeding continues, it is called internal hemorrhage. If the bleeding is 200 mL of blood per hour via the intercostal tube then it is considered large hemothorax.

Surgery

The surgery is performed using endotracheal anesthesia combined with muscle relaxants. The incision is made in between 5th and 6th intercostal space and the chest is opened. The pleural cavity is cleared from blood fibrin. Blood fibrin covers the lungs that prevents the full lung inflation. Once blood fibrin is removed the lung will start to reexpand then the incision is closed and water sealed bottle drainage is connected and continues until radiograph is taken and lung expansion is completely seen.

▎LUNG CONTUSION AND LACERATION

Lung is the intrathoracic organ and is most commonly injured. Lung contusion or pulmonary contusion is lung bruise. It leads to blood, fluids, and capillaries damage leading to lung tissue accumulation. Excess fluid causes gas exchange interference leading to hypoxia.

Causes

1. Pneumothorax
2. Hemothorax
3. Pulmonary contusion
4. Pulmonary hematoma
5. Systemic air emboli
6. Acute respiratory distress syndrome
7. Chest trauma
8. Explosives
9. Road traffic accident

Clinical Features

1. Chest pain
2. Cyanosis
3. Coughing blood

Complications

1. Continued hemothorax of >1,500 mL
2. Massive air leak
3. Development of nonhealing lung abscess
4. Pulmonary necrosis
5. Pulmonary edema
6. Pneumonia
7. Acute respiratory distress syndrome
8. Hemorrhage in alveoli

Diagnosis

1. Physical examination
2. Chest radiography

Treatment

1. Supplement oxygen
2. ICU treatment
3. Tube thoracotomy
4. Mechanical ventilation for patients with compromised breathing
5. Fluid replacement for adequate blood volume if fluid overloaded then leading to pulmonary edema
6. Pneumorrhaphy

7. Suturing
8. Stapling

Physical Therapy Management

Same as of Fracture (Refer page 124).

PULMONARY LACERATION

The pulmonary laceration occurs when lung tissue is cut leading to pulmonary hematoma and collection of blood in the lung tissue. The collapsed lung occurs with hemothorax, pneumothorax, and hemopneumothorax.

Clinical Features

Low oxygen saturation, cyanosis, dyspnea, painful breathing, decreased exercise tolerance, rapid breathing, and rapid heart rate.

Treatment

The pulmonary laceration condition is treated using supplemental oxygen, ventilation, thoracotomy tube is used to removed air and blood from the chest cavity.

Physical Therapy Management

Same as of Fracture (Refer page 124).

INJURY TO HEART, GREAT VESSELS, AND BRONCHUS

1. Rupture of aorta
2. Ascending aorta/main pulmonary artery injury
3. Aortic arch-thoracic outlet vascular injury, distal innominate artery, and vein
4. Subclavian vascular injury
5. Descending thoracic aorta
6. Bronchial injury
7. Penetrating cardiac injury
8. Stab wound of heart
9. Coronary artery injury

Rupture of Aorta

It is a fatal injury. A part of the arch of the aorta which lies distal to the origin of the left subclavian artery near its junction with the descending aorta is affected by injury. Aorta is the largest artery and when the aorta ruptures it leads to dangerous condition. Secondary to aorta supplies blood to systemic circulation. The common causes are abdominal aortic aneurysm. The inner wall of aorta is tore and can block the blood flow to the heart and abdominal organs.

Causes

Cardiac surgery, trauma, ruptured aortic aneurysm and vascular surgery.

Clinical Features

Back pain, abdominal pain, flank pain, loss of consciousness, fast heart rate or tachycardia, cyanosis, low blood pressure leading to hypovolemic shock, altered mental status, retroperitoneal bleeding, and death.

Diagnosis

- **X-ray:** Widening of the mediastinum due to accumulation of blood
- **Aortography:** This provides the actual site of injury to aorta.
- Computed tomography (CT) scan and ultrasound.

Complications

1. Shock
2. Anemia
3. Brain ischemia
4. Spinal cord ischemia

Prevention

Screening for aortic disease.

Treatment

Open repair of aortic disease for nonruptured aortic aneurysm, endovascular therapy, endovascular aneurysm repair (EVAR), aortic occlusion using balloon to stabilize the patient to prevent blood loss before anesthesia is given.

Ascending Aorta Injury

The injury to portion of aorta lies in chest cavity.

Anatomy

It is the first section of aorta. It starts from left ventricle of heart to aortic arch. Its total length is 5 cm or 2 inches. It gives rise to two branches. They are right coronary artery (CA) and left CA. The size of artery if 3.5 cm or greater called dilated ascending aorta and if the size is 4.5 cm then it is indicative of thoracic aortic aneurysm. The standard size is 4.3 cm in elderly population. The ascending aortic and pulmonary artery are enclosed in pericardium. Ascending aorta is covered by trunk of pulmonary artery.

This occurs due to trauma of ascending aorta leading to disruption or transection.

Pathology

Aorta gets compressed between structures such as clavicle, first rib, manubrium, and spine. In ascending aorta, the cause is torsion. It is a two-way twisting of the aorta. Porcelain aorta is atherosclerosis of ascending aorta.

Cause

Gunshot injury.

Types

- Laceration or tear
- **Transection:** Axis or cross section
- Rupture is the forcible disruption of the ascending aorta tissue and is of two types partial and complete.

Complication

Pericardial tamponade and death.

Treatment

1. Thoracotomy
2. Cardiopulmonary bypass with reconstruction
3. Surgery causes aortic embolism and aortic injury.

Main Pulmonary Artery Injury

This artery helps for pulmonary circulation. It carries deoxygenated blood from heart to lungs on right side of heart.

Types

It is of two types:
1. Large main pulmonary artery or pulmonary trunk that comes from the heart
2. Small pulmonary artery has branches to arterioles, capillaries, and pulmonary alveoli.

Pulmonary Trunk

Main pulmonary artery or pulmonary trunk is at the base of right ventricle. It divides into right and left main pulmonary artery. Right main pulmonary artery is longer and divided into truncus anterior that supplies right upper lobe and interlobar artery supplies middle and lower lobe of the lung. The left pulmonary artery divides into lobar arteries for each lobe of the lung. Right and left main pulmonary arteries give branches to lobar artery to segmental artery, subsegmental pulmonary artery, and interlobular artery.

Functions

This carries deoxygenated blood from right ventricle to lungs then to capillaries and to alveoli and gets oxygenated and supplies to the whole body. It is part of respiration process.

Clinical Significance

Pulmonary artery hypertension is increase pressure > 25 mm Hg.

Diagnosis

Computed tomography scan: It shows evaluation of pulmonary trunk injury, lung parenchyma, soft tissue injury.

Pulmonary Embolism

Embolism in pulmonary circulation due to deep vein thrombosis (DVT) causing death in cancer and stroke patients. Large embolism goes to right and left main pulmonary artery called saddle embolism. Pulmonary artery pressure is measured by using catheter in main pulmonary artery. There are two types of pressure. They are—mean pressure is about 9-18 mm Hg and wedge pressure is about 6-12 mm Hg. This increases in left ventricle heart failure and mitral valve stenosis.

Aortic Arch—Thoracic Outlet Vascular Injury, Distal Innominate Artery, and Vein

Aortic Arch Injury

Rupture or torn of the aorta is fatal because the injury causes fatal bleeding. As aorta supplies blood to the whole body, the blood pressure is high. Any tear or rupture causes loss of blood rapidly leading to shock and death. Aortic rupture is caused by abdominal aortic aneurysm.

Clinical features
Dyspnea, back pain, dysphagia, upper and lower body blood pressure varies with high upper body pressure measure in upper extremity and low lower body pressure measured with lower extremity, cough, chest pain.

Diagnosis
Radiograph shows wide mediastinum, left hemothorax, CT angiogram is also done as one of the diagnostic measure. Renal failure causes decreased urine output, increased creatine levels.

Treatment
Medical treatment: Beta-blockers and vasodilators to decrease blood pressure.

Surgical treatment: Aortic transection is the surgical treatment for this condition and complication of this surgery would be paraplegia, endovascular repair.

Ascending Aortic Rupture

Ascending aorta is the first section of aorta. It starts from left ventricle of heart to aortic arch. The total length is 5 cm or 2 inches..

Ascending aortic branches to right CA and left CA. Both supplies blood to the heart muscle. The size of aorta when dilated is 3.5 cm and greater and if there is presence of thoracic aortic aneurysm then size would be 4.5 cm. In elderly, the size would be 4.3 cm which is the standard size.

The ascending aorta and pericardium are enclosed in pericardium and ascending aorta is covered by trunk of pulmonary artery.

Clinical features
Porcelain aorta is atherosclerosis of ascending aorta.

Traumatic aorta rupture or thoracic aorta disruption or transection. It is injury to the portion of aorta.

Causes
1. Pathology
2. **Trauma:** It can be deceleration injury such as car accident and falls from height and crush injury.

Pathology
The aorta gets compressed between structures such as clavicle, first rib manubrium, and spine. In ascending aorta the cause is torsion. It is a two-way twisting.

Classification
Ascending aortic rupture is classified into three types:
1. Laceration or tear
2. Transection or cross section
3. Rupture is disruption of tissue. It is of two types. They are partial and complete.

Treatment
Surgery is the treatment for this condition and complications for this surgery could be aortic embolism and aortic injury.

Descending Thoracic Aorta Injury

This is a lethal injury.

Causes

Penetrating or blunt trauma causing rapid deceleration during rapid high speed accident or fall from height.

Clinical Features

The descending aorta remains in the place due to mediastinal pleural fixation and causes tear of descending thoracic aorta at the origin of the left subclavian artery.

Prognosis

The patient is seen with multisystem injury and dies at the site of the accident or during emergency resuscitation.

Main Pulmonary Artery Injury

This artery helps for pulmonary circulation. It carries deoxygenated blood from heart to lungs on the right side.

Types

It is divided into large and small arteries. The *large artery* is main pulmonary artery or pulmonary trunk that comes from the heart and the *small arteries* are arterioles divided into capillaries around pulmonary alveoli.

Pulmonary trunk
The main pulmonary artery or pulmonary trunk at the base of right ventricle is divided into right main pulmonary artery and left main pulmonary artery. The left artery is divided into lobar arteries for each lobe of the left lung.

Right main pulmonary artery
It is divided into truncus anterior and supplies to right upper extremity and interlobar artery is divided into medial lobe of lung and inner lobe of lungs.

Right and left main pulmonary artery is divided into lobar artery, then to segmental artery, then to subsegmental pulmonary artery, and finally into intralobular artery.

Functions

The main function of the pulmonary trunk is to carry deoxygenated blood from right ventricle to lungs and from lungs to capillaries to alveoli where blood gets oxygenated and via four pulmonary veins enter left atrium to left ventricle through aorta goes into systemic circulation.

Clinical Significance

Pulmonary artery hypertension is increased pressure > 25 mm Hg.

Diagnosis

Computed tomography scan shows evaluation of pulmonary trunk injury, lung parenchyma, soft tissue injury. If diameter is >29 mm Hg, it indicates pulmonary hypertension that can lead to heart failure, COPD and scleroderma.

The thrombus is formed and when it travels called embolus and when the embolus travels in pulmonary circulation is called pulmonary embolism. This can lead to death. This is a serious condition. Immediate diagnosis and treatment should be done or it turns out to be fatal.

Thoracic Outlet Vascular Injury

Vascular Thoracic Outlet Syndrome

- **Thoracic outlet:** The thoracic outlet is the pathway for brachial plexus, subclavian artery and subclavian vein in between first rib and clavicle.
- **Borders:** There are four borders for thoracic outlet
- **Anterior border:** Formed by clavicle, pectoralis minor
- **Posterior border:** Upper trapezius and scapula
- **Medial border:** Scalene muscles like anterior, medial and posterior
- **Lateral border:** Axilla
- **Thoracic outlet syndrome:** This is the syndrome where compression of blood vessels and nerves are seen.

Types

The four types of compression are arteries, veins [vascular thoracic outlet syndrome (TOS)], nerves, and nonspecific TOS.

1. Arterial TOS is compression is subclavian artery compression under the clavicle.
2. Venous TOS is compression is subclavian vein compression under the clavicle.
3. Neurogenic TOS is compression of brachial plexus nerves.
4. Nonspecific TOS or disputed TOS: The main clinical feature of this type is chronic pain in thoracic outlet and increases with activity but the causes of the pain is not determined.

Types of Thoracic Outlet Syndrome

1. Scalene syndrome
2. Costoclavicular syndrome
3. Pectoralis syndrome
4. Hyperabduction syndrome
5. Droopy shoulder syndrome

Scalene syndrome: The syndrome occurs due to compression of structures between scalene muscles and first rib. The scalene muscles are hypertrophied or tight causing compression of the proximal portion of the brachial plexus.

Diagnosis: Adson Test.

The physical therapist (PT) locates radial pulse. The head is rotated to the same side. Head is extended. The PT lateral rotates and extend the patient shoulder. The patient is asked to take deep breath and hold the breath. The PT notices the pulse disappears or decreased with subclavian artery compression and the test is considered positive.

Costoclavicular syndrome: The costoclavicular space is in between clavicle and first rib. The cause of the syndrome is carrying heavy suitcase, carrying heavy shoulder bag, faulty posture like forward head, increased thoracic kyphosis, protracted scapula and forward shoulders. The muscles that are short are scalene, pectoralis major, levator scapulae and subscapularis, 1st rib subluxation, upper thoracic breathing seen in conditions like chronic emphysema and asthma, also using accessory muscles like serratus anterior, levator scapulae.

Diagnosis: Military Brace Test: The physical therapist palpates radial pulse, the shoulder is brought down and back patient is asked to look forward slightly rotating the head to opposite side.

Pectoralis syndrome: The cause of this syndrome is compression occurring between pectoralis minor muscle and coracoid process. The causes can be faulty posture, pectoralis minor muscle tightness causing scapula to tip forward.

Diagnosis: Roos Test or Elevated Arm Stress Test: The patient stand abduct the arm to 90. Lateral rotate, elbow flexion to 90. Patient open and closes hand for three minutes. If the patient gets ischemic pain, heaviness, weakness, numbness and tingling. The test is considered positive if the patient unable to hold the initial position.

Hyperabduction syndrome: The patient will have thoracic outlet syndrome.

Diagnosis: Wright Test: Sitting: The physical therapist locates the pulse, the shoulder moves to abduction and external rotation and patient asked to take deep breath and rotate the head to opposite site. If the symptoms increase then test is considered positive.

Allen Maneuver: The patient is in sitting. The upper limb is abducted 90 degrees, elbow flexion and external rotation. Patient is asked to take a deep breath and rotate the head to opposite side and if symptoms increases then test is positive.

Droopy shoulder symptoms: The patient has throacic outlet syndrome symptoms secondary to depression of the shoulder that stretches brachial plexus that causes pain. The cause of this can be imbalance between weak and tight muscles and over us of one side muscles, sleeping on one side.

Causes

Baseball injury, repetitive overhead motion and swimming. Trauma is caused by clavicle fracture, repetitive is nonergonomic posture, athletics such as swimming, badminton, and dancers. The population affected is athletics and young patients.

1. **Arterial thoracic outlet syndrome**: It is compression of subclavian artery. The subclavian artery is the branch of aortic arch and travels along brachial plexus, between scalene muscles (anterior and middle scalene) over the first rib and under clavicle.
   Clinical features: Thromboembolism is clot formation and dislodging which causes distal ischemia in the part of the hand, arm fatigue, stroke and Raynaud's phenomenon. Repetitive overhead activities causes subclavian artery compression with arm movement. The causes can be long C7 transverse process, cervical rib, clavicle fracture, first rib articulation, and rib fracture.
   Diagnosis: CT angiogram, MR (magnetic resonance) angiogram or conventional angiography, physical examination, and the imaging are done with arm placing above the head so can access for active compression of subclavian artery.
   Treatment: Surgical removal of the cause reduces symptoms from soft tissue or bone, repair of subclavian artery, repair of aneurysm (bulging of arterial wall), occlusion of the artery (can be partial or complete ischemia). Sympathectomy is the treatment.

2. **Venous thoracic outlet syndrome**: Paget-Schroetter syndrome or subclavian vein effort thrombosis:
   Clinical features: The subclavian vein thrombosis occurs due to arm swelling.

3. **Neurogenic thoracic outlet syndrome:** It is the compression of the brachial plexus. The brachial plexus is network of the nerves arising from spinal cord. Brachial plexus controls sensory sensation of the upper extremity and motor control of the muscles of upper extremity.
   Clinical features: Weak grip muscles, tingling or numbness in the arm or fingers is seen.
   Gilliatt-Sumner hand: This condition is muscle wasting of the thumb. Other symptoms are pain in the hand, shoulder, and neck.

4. **Non-specific thoracic outlet syndrome or disputed thoracic outlet syndrome:** The main clinical feature of this type is chronic pain. Pain in the thoracic outlet that increases with activity but the cause of the pain cannot be determined.

Thoracic Surgery

Causes
The causes of all types of TOS are as follows:
1. **Pregnancy:** The signs of TOS can be seen secondary to loosened joints.
2. **Anatomical defects:** It is congenital defect by birth like having a cervical rib. It is the extra rib above the first rib and tight band that is abnormal and connects the rib to the spine.
3. **Repetitive activity:** Using computer, lifting above the head such as stocking the shelves, athletes such as swimmer and baseball pitcher, trauma such as car accident, pressure in obesity and carrying backpack, poor posture such as forward head and shoulder dropping.

Risk factors
Age: 20–40 years,
Sex: Female

Complications
Early diagnosis can be treated with conservative management but if delayed leads to complication and surgical treatment is the only left option.

Prevention
The condition should be treated early as it may lead to permanent damage; if overweight then losing weight is the option, if susceptible to the condition avoid lifting heavy objects and repetitive movement.

Perform daily exercises, stretching, strengthening muscles of shoulder, neck, and chest.

Diagnosis
- **Physical examination:** Shoulder depression, abnormal pulse, limited range of motion, swelling in arm.
- **Medical examination:** Physical activity and examination.

Treatment
If the condition is diagnosed early then treatment options would be medications and physical therapy management.

Physical therapy management for thoracic outlet syndrome

S. No.	Aims of physical therapy	Plans of physical therapy
1.	To stretch the short muscles	Muscles like scalene, levator scapula, subscapularis and pectoralis minor

Contd...

Contd...

S. No.	Aims of physical therapy	Plans of physical therapy
2.	To stretch muscles according to the syndrome affected	*Scalene syndrome:* Stretch scalene *Costoclavicular syndrome:* Postural reeducation *Axillary or pectoralis minor syndrome:* Stretch pectoralis minor *Droopy shoulder syndrome:* Emphasize on using both sides
3.	Mobilize restricted neurological tissue	Nerve mobilization
4.	Mobilize restricted joint, connective tissue, muscle structures	Stretching is performed
5.	To correct faulty breathing pattern	Use of upper thorax should be avoided and avoid use of accessory muscles of respiration like scalene, levator scapulae, serratus anterior and pectoralis minor
6.	Teach proper breathing pattern	Relax upper thorax, encourage abdominal breathing
7.	To train functional independence	Patient awareness about signs and symptoms, precautions, dos and don'ts. Home exercise program

Bronchial Injury

It is the injury to airway structures that includes bronchi and trachea also called tracheobronchial injury.

Location

Right and left stem bronchus.

Causes

1. Injury to chest or neck can be penetrating or blunt trauma.
2. Iatrogenic occurs during intubation, tracheostomy, and bronchoscopy.
3. Inhalation of smoke.
4. Aspiration of liquids and objects.

Clinical Features

Dyspnea, respiratory distress, dysphonia, coughing, rapid breathing, hemoptysis, abnormal breath sounds.

Types

This is of two types:
1. Disruption of pleura causing pneumothorax
2. Nondisruption of pleura.

Prevention

Wearing seat belt during travel.

Diagnosis

Radiography finding shows airway wall irregularities, tracheal wall or bronchial wall thickening, laryngeal wall disruption.

Computed tomography or CT scan findings help to visualize tracheobronchial tree.

Prognosis

Life-threatening respiratory insufficiency.

Treatment

Emergency care such as tracheal intubation so that airway would remain open and if required, surgery is performed. Mortality rate is 30%.

Treatment might be difficult as prognosis is poor but early diagnosis can prevent complications such as respiratory tract infection, damage to the lung tissue and stenosis of the airway. The treatment is done by using supplemental oxygen and mechanical ventilation.

Complications

Pneumonia, sepsis, multiple organ dysfunction syndrome, atelectasis, subcutaneous emphysema.

Late complications are pneumonia and bronchiectasis.

Penetrating Cardiac Injury

The penetrating cardiac injury causes injury to vital organs such as lungs and heart that interfere with breathing and circulation.

Site

Coronary arteries are most commonly injured.

Causes

Penetrating object pierces through the skin and enters the body tissue and creates an open wound whereas non-penetrating or blunt trauma intact skin may or may not be present. Some common examples are gunshot injury, stabbing injury when there is serious injury causes complications like infection and shock.

Diagnosis

Radiograph and CT scan.

Treatment

Repair of the arteries and removal of the foreign object is required.

Complications

Spinal motion restriction is seen after surgery.

Lung Injury or Pulmonary Laceration or Contusion

Pulmonary contusion is cut in the lung's tissues and pulmonary laceration is bruise in the lung tissue.

Types
- **Pneumothorax:** Air in the chest cavity outside the lung
- **Hemothorax:** Blood in the chest cavity outside the lung.
- **Hemopneumothorax:** Air and blood in the chest cavity outside the lungs.
- **Heart injury:** Profuse bleeding to chest cavity.
- **Pericardial or cardiac tamponade:** This condition is when the fluid in the pericardium increases causing compression of the heart.

Stab Injury of Heart

Stab injury is trauma to the skin by a sharp object such as knife. Stab injury leads to external and internal injuries. Heart injury and abdominal injury are common.

Causes

Large hole in the heart.

Clinical Features

1. Hemothorax
2. Pericardial tamponade

Diagnosis

Computed tomography scan, contrast studies, internal bleeding is diagnosed using diagnostic peritoneal lavage (DPL), focused assessment with sonography for trauma (FAST).
Lab test: WBC, hematocrit and liver function tests.

Treatment

Depending upon the severity of injury the treatment is done. The options of treatment are airway management, control of hemorrhage, shock management. Most important aspect is to maintain vital signs like body temperature and systolic blood pressure. Surgical treatment is done if the extent of injury is large.

Complication

Laceration of artery causes death.

Coronary Artery Injury

The CA injury is uncommon but it is very dangerous because coronary artery supply is cut-off causing hematoma in arterial wall leading to weak artery wall. Spontaneous CA dissection leads to heart attack.

Causes

During and after pregnancy, connective tissue disorder such as Marfan syndrome.

Clinical Features

Shortness of breath, chest pain, sweating, rapid heartbeat, nausea, dizziness, extreme tiredness, cardiogenic shock, ventricular arrhythmia, radiating pain along left arm, left side of neck, pain in the upper abdomen, and sudden cardiac death.

Pathophysiology

Injury to the layers of arterial wall leads to formation of hematoma. Hematoma forms false lumen that restricts the true lumen leading to restriction of blood flow to the heart muscles, limited oxygen and nutrients supply to the myocardium. All these causes ischemia and death of the myocardium leading to the heart attack or myocardial infarction.

Diagnosis

- **ECG:** ST-elevation

- **Angiography:** False lumen and true lumen differentiation
- **Intracoronary imaging:** Distinguish injury from atherosclerosis

Treatment

Depends upon the clinical features, severity of injury, and complications.

The following treatment options are available. They are rib resection, decortication and window operation.

EMPYEMA

Definition

It is the collection of the pus in existing anatomical cavity. Abscess is the collection of pus in a newly formed cavity. Pleural empyema occurs in pleural cavity by bacteria.

Causes

Pneumonia, chest cavity and chest injury.

Clinical Features

Cough, fever, shortness of breath and chest pain.

Pathology

When there is pleural infection, there is a serious effusion causing inflammatory changes, exudation of fluid, fibrin deposits, intrapleural clotting all leading to empyema. There is a fusion of lung to chest wall at the periphery. There is a collection of fluid, formation of granulation tissue, plaques of fibrous tissue, and adhesions are formed. The fluid becomes thick and empyema is localized. A mature empyema consists of visceral and parietal layers of the fibrous tissue on the lung. The fibrous tissue contracts, the ribs are drawn together and lose their mobility. The diaphragm is elevated and fixed, mediastinum is drawn towards the affected side. Lung becomes immobile and functionless called chronic empyema or frozen chest.

Stages

There are three stages of empyema:
1. **Exudative stage:** In this stage, there is increase of pleural fluid with pus or no pus and swelling of pleural membranes.
2. **Fibrinopurulent stage:** In this stage, the pus pockets are formed with fibrous septa and fibrin deposit occurs.

3. **Organizing stage:** Lung scarring leads to loss of ability to expand, fibroblasts grow and collagen deposit occurs.

Diagnosis

Chest radiograph and ultrasound: To know the collection of pleural fluid and size of cavity. Chest CT and MRI, blood and sputum culture.

Treatment

1. To control infection: Antibiotics treatment
2. Evacuation of pus: Pleural fluid drainage or chest tube drainage
3. Obliteration of pleural space
4. Re-expansion of lung: Chest PT
5. Restoration of normal pulmonary function antibiotics

Prognosis

Resident needs follow-up with repeatable chest X-ray after 4 weeks of discharge from hospital. It returns to normal by 6 months. Long-term pleural empyema causes bronchopleural fistula formation, pleural thickening, recurrent empyema leading to lungs impairment that requires surgical decortication.

Types of Empyema

Empyema is classified as three types: (1) Acute empyema, (2) Sub-acute empyema, and (3) Chronic empyema.

1. Acute Empyema

Causes
1. Secondary to pulmonary infection, e.g., pneumonia.
2. Infective process, e.g., TB, lung abscess, and bronchiectasis.
3. Inflammatory conditions, e.g., osteomyelitis of rib, osteomyelitis of dorsal spine.
4. Trauma: Perforation of esophagus and rupture of lung abscess.
5. Spontaneous pneumothorax.
6. Iatrogenic.

Clinical features
1. Toxemia
2. Shock with pleural pain
3. Rapid hallow breathing

Diagnosis
Needle exploration confirms signs of pleural fluid.

Treatment
1. Early thoracotomy is required.
2. Pus aspiration on alternate days.
3. Antibiotics to control the infection.
4. Intercostal tube drainage if aspiration failed. Intercostal catheter inserted through a cannula and connected to an under-water seal.

2. Sub-acute Empyema

The sub-acute empyema develops suddenly.

Clinical features
1. Fever
2. Pneumonia
3. Diminished chest movement
4. Dullness
5. Absent breath sounds
6. Displacement of viscera

Causes
1. Empyema of >3 months duration
2. Mismanagement of one and two stages of empyema
3. Failure to diagnose the original condition
4. Complication of an underlying condition of lung, bronchiectasis, lung abscess, and tumor
5. Foreign bodies
6. Actionomycosis
7. Chronic infection
8. Carcinoma lung
9. Bronchopleural fistula
10. Inadequate drainage of subphrenic abscess.

The other types of empyema are:
1. **Latent empyema:** A closed collection of pus separated from its surrounding.
2. **Bronchopleural fistula:** Empyema discharging continuous or intermittently into a bronchus.
3. **Persistent empyema:** Empyema discharging continuous or intermittently through a sinus in chest wall.

Symptoms
1. Pleuritic chest pain
2. Heavy sensation on the side
3. Fever
4. Dyspnea

5. Tachycardia
6. Cough with purulent sputum
7. Decreased chest exertion
8. Pain on percussion
9. Friction rub
10. Absent blood supply

Complications
1. Chronicity
2. Septicemia
3. Rupture of bronchus
4. Metastasis abscess in vertebrae and brain
5. Pyopneumothorax
6. Empyema necessitans

Diagnosis
1. Exploration of pus by needle.
2. Iodized oil should be injected into the empyema to locate the lowest point and to know which rib has to be resected.

Treatment
1. Rib resection:
Indication
- When conservative method fails because of infection by resistant organism
- Loculated empyema
- Bronchopleural fistula or esophageal fistula
- Bronchiectasis or tumor

Procedure
The surgery is carried under local anesthesia. An oblique incision is made through the skin over the rib to be resected. The periosteum of the rib is elevated by 5 cm and segment is exercised. The rib bed is incised. Care needs to be taken to avoid damage to the intercostal vessels. The opening is enlarged to permit complete evacuation of the empyema. Inspection through biopsy of the pleura should be done. Drainage should be closed at first using an underwater seal. If drainage gets reduced to 60 mL daily, open drainage should be started. The drainage should be maintained till the empyema cavity gets completely obliterated which takes as long as 6–8 weeks. If the tube is removed prematurely, it leads to chronicity of the condition. Regular investigations are done using serial pleurogram with radio-opaque oil injected into the empyema cavity at an interval of 3 weeks. The projection of tube should be 2.5–5 cm into the empyema cavity initially,

which is later adjusted to 4 cm. The intercostal drainage is connected if pus is present. Patient should attend postoperative physical therapy session for early recovery, prevent complication and getting back to prior level of function. Thus physical therapy plays an important role.

2. Decortication:

Definition
This surgery is removal of the cortex or external covering from any organ or structure along with the removal of the thickened pleura.

Procedure
Patient is in the lateral position. An incision is made in the 5th intercostal space. The blood clots are removed and any adhesions between the parietal and visceral pleura are divided. The anesthesiologist inflates lung to know the site and extent of entrapment by the fibrinous membrane over the visceral pleura. The lungs are deflated slightly, the incision is made transversely or longitudinally and separation of the peel is done. The peel may vary from a fraction of a millimeter to several cm in thickness. The lung bulges once visceral pleura is reached through the incision. The edges of the incision are elevated and separated. Fingertip is inserted and separated rapidly. If hemothorax is present for many weeks or months or when decortication is done for chronic empyema, then the membrane may be adherent to the visceral pleura and sharp dissection is required. The entire visceral membrane is removed, then lung expands completely and parietal membrane is also removed.

Lung expansion is maintained during the postoperative period to prevent the recurrence. There are 2 to 3 drainage tubes are inserted and constant suction is performed. Air leaks may persist for several days when multiple injuries to the superior alveoli are present.

3. Chronic Empyema

It is chronic stage of empyema. The duration of empyema is for 3 months or more.

The treatment option for chronic empyema is window operation or open flap procedure. Eloesser introduced in 1935.

Indication
1. Unsuccessful open drainage
2. Improper closed drainage

Uses
1. Chronic empyema
2. Drain post-pneumonectomy empyema.

Procedure

The u-shaped flap of skin is made with a base of 10–12 cm long and parallel to the superior border of the first uninvolved rib above the bottom of the empyema cavity. The full curved end of the flap is 6–7 cm long, the rib underlying the base of the flap is resected, turned into chest and taken to pleura. The skin defect is allowed to heal by secondary intention.

Pulmonary rehabilitation program: Same as of pneumothorax (Refer page 131).

PULMONARY TUBERCULOSIS

Definition

It is the disease caused by *Mycobacterium tuberculosis*. The bacteria attacks lungs and other parts of the body. Tuberculosis is an airborne disease which spreads through air when the individual cough, sneezes or talks.

Types

Tuberculosis is classified into two categories. They are:
1. Latent
2. Active tuberculosis.

Latent Tuberculosis

Resident has TB infection but bacteria are in inactive stage with no symptoms. This type can turn into active TB so treatment is important.

Active Tuberculosis

The first few weeks of active tuberculosis is a airborne infection. The patient is very sick and spreads the germs easily so mandatory isolation of the patient with medical treatment is necessary.

Clinical Features

Active Tuberculosis

Loss of appetite, chills, weight loss, blood containing mucus, fever, night sweats, coughing, fatigue, chest pain, nail clubbing. Tuberculosis spreads by air on exposure with person having active TB when they sneeze, spit, cough, or speak. The active disease of tuberculosis is seen in individual with HIV/AIDS and cigarette smokers.

Types of Tuberculosis

Location of tuberculosis is of two types—pulmonary and extrapulmonary tuberculosis.

Pulmonary Tuberculosis

This is active TB of the lungs and symptoms are cough producing sputum, chest pain. This is seen in upper lobe of lungs secondary to decreased lymphatic drainage, if the infection spreads to pulmonary artery then it causes massive bleeding.

Extrapulmonary Tuberculosis

It occurs in persons with weak immune system. The sites are TB affecting pleura (TB pleurisy), lymphatic system TB (scrofula of the neck), genitourinary system (urogenital TB), bones, and joints: Pott's disease of spine, disseminated TB, or miliary. The most fatal tuberculosis of all extrapulmonary tuberculosis is miliary tuberculosis.

Complications

Early

Pneumonia, empyema, hemoptysis, laryngitis and pneumothorax.

Late Complications

Bronchiectasis, mycetomes in cavities, colonization of fibrotic lung with nontuberculous mycobacterium, nonrespiratory disease, bone disease and genitourinary disease.

Diagnosis

- **Active TB:** Chest X-ray, sputum culture
- **Latent TB:** Tuberculin skin test/Mantoux tuberculin test and blood tests.

Radiograph

Snow storm appearance, cavity formation and calcification are seen.

Tuberculin Test

This test should be done within 6 weeks of infection.

Treatment

Antibiotics, MDR-TB (multiple drug-resistant TB), XDR-TB (extensively drug-resistant TB).

Active Tuberculosis

Antibiotic treatment is given to reduce the infection and also decrease the risk of developing resistance to the drugs.

Latent Tuberculosis

Isoniazid and rifampicin for 3 months to prevent progression to active TB, 6 months antibiotics such as rifampicin, isoniazid, pyrazinamide, ethambutol for 2 months. Rifampicin and isoniazid for the last 4 months. If bacterial resistance is high to drug isoniazid, then alternative drug is ethambutol.

Recurrent disease: If TB recurs, then drug resistance test is done to know about the antibiotic sensitivity. If multiple drug resistance is confirmed, the treatment will be given with four antibiotics for 18 to 24 months.

Prevention

1. High-risk people who are screening for disease can be vaccinated with BCG (bacillus Calmette-Guerin).
2. Pasteurization of milk prevents transmission of the tubercle to humans from cow's milk.
3. Sputum must be disposed carefully to avoid cross infection.
4. The doctors, physical therapist, nurses and all health-care workers who are more prone for the droplet infection needs to take precaution.

POTT'S DISEASE/POTT'S PARAPLEGIA/POTT'S SPINE/TUBERCULOSIS SPONDYLITIS

Definition

Pott's spine is the TB of the vertebra. The most commonly affected areas are upper lumbar and lower thoracic vertebra.

Causes

It occurs as a result of hematogenous spread from lungs to adjacent vertebra to intervertebral disk space. The disk becomes avascular and devoid of nutrients therefore collapses causing caseous necrosis leading to death of the disk tissue, vertebral narrowing, spinal damage, and vertebral collapse.

Clinical Features

Neurological defects leads to spinal cord compression such as paresis, nerve root pain, paraplegia, impaired sensation, cauda equina syndrome.

Spinal deformity leading to kyphosis, muscle spasm, restricted spinal motion, localized tenderness. Back pain is the earliest symptom with radicular or spinal pain, fever, malaise, night sweat, and weight loss. Cervical spinal TB is seen in 10% of affected population. The clinical features are severe neurological complications such as pain, stiffness, hoarseness, torticollis, hemiplegia or quadriplegia.

TB spine is common with HIV.

Pott's Disease Systemic Involvement

The systems affected are musculoskeletal, neurological, cardiovascular, integumentary, urogenital, and other symptoms.
1. Vertebral fracture, paresthesia, spinal artery infection, pressure ulcer, bowel dysfunction and fever
2. Vertebral collapse, paralysis of lower extremity depending on the spinal level affected, decreased vascularity to intervertebral discs, abscess formation, rupture of abscess, bladder dysfunction and night sweat are seen
3. Destruction of spinal ligament: Paresis, thrombosis, fungal infection, and malaise
4. IV disk destruction, abnormal muscle tone, weight loss
5. Abscess—abnormal reflex
6. Osteoporosis, osteopenia—cauda equina syndrome
7. Dislocated vertebra
8. Muscle atrophy
9. Kyphotic deformity
10. Torticollis

Diagnosis

- ESR is elevated. The rate is >100 mm/h
- Tuberculin skin test is positive
- CBC, leukocytosis

- Radiographic images shows increased anterior wedging, destruction of anterior portion of the vertebral body, sclerosis, collapse of vertebral body, osteoporotic vertebral end-plates, bone lesions occur at more than one level, intervertebral disk shrink, abscess formation, vertebral body destruction
- Bone scan: Shows nerve compression, disk space infection
- MRI shows osteomyelitis of spine
- Bone biopsy
- Computed tomography scan: Disk collapse, bone circumference disruption, early lesions, soft tissue abscess

Prevention

The main goal is to prevent the spread of the infection for the individuals who tested positive for purified protein derivative (PPD) test, positive chest radiograph by prescribing effective medication treatment.

Treatment

It is divided into three types.

Conservative Treatment

Anti-TB medication, analgesics, spine mobilization using braces and collars depending on affected site.

Surgical Treatment

Draining spinal abscess, decompression of spinal cord, stabilizing the spine, full debridement of bony lesions so requires spinal fusion at thoracic level with or without instrumentation. Posterior fusion decreases kyphosis with anterior approach, severe kyphotic deformity >30 needs posterior approach.

Physical Therapy Treatment

Modalities to reduce the pain such as TENS, postural reeducation exercises, strengthening and flexibility of trunk muscles, and home exercise program.
- **Spinal decompression:** Spinal stabilization exercises, back strengthening exercises, Maitland techniques.
- **Spinal fusion:** Transcutaneous electrical nerve stimulation (TENS) for neuropathic pain, walking program, trunk strengthening, aerobic exercise, and aquatic therapy.

Complications

Spinal cord compression leads to paraplegia, vertebral collapse leads to kyphosis, sinus formation.

Prognosis

Good prognosis is seen in younger age group, partial spinal cord compression, early onset with delayed neurological complications and shorter duration of the complications.

Pulmonary rehabilitation program: Same as of pneumothorax (Refer page 131).

▌TUBERCULOMA

The tuberculoma is the tubercles form into lump with calcification. It is one of the TB clinical manifestation.

Causes

TB bacteria forms calcium crystals and effects lungs, brain, ovaries, esophagus, intestine, bones, liver, and pancreas.

Clinical Features

Raised intracranial pressure causes headache, impairment of conscious level, papilledema, vomiting, bradycardia, and arterial hypertension.

Diagnosis

- Computed tomography angiography (CTA).
- Nuclear magnetic resonance imaging (NMRI): This is a procedure where detailed pictures of areas inside the body are created and also shows difference between normal and diseased areas.
- Erythrocyte sedimentation rate (ESR): It is one of the diagnostic test done during initial stages of tuberculosis. The normal rate is 1-13 mm/hr in men and 1-20 mm/hr in women. In tuberculosis the ESR is very high, greater than 100 mm/hr.
- X-ray chest.
- Tuberculin test.

Management

1. Antituberculous therapy such as HRZE. It is group of four medications used in combination as antibiotic treatment for

tuberculosis. H is Isoniazid, R is Rifampicin, Z is Pyrazinamide and E is Ethambutol
2. Measures to relieve intracranial tension
3. Surgical excision of tumor mass.

Pulmonary rehabilitation program: Same as of pneumothorax (Refer page 131).

BRONCHIECTASIS SICCA

Definition

Bronchiectasis sicca also called dry bronchiectasis is a rare form of bronchiectasis. It is a chronic permanent dilatation of the bronchi with impaired damage of secretions and recurrent lower respiratory tract infection. It is a dry form of the bronchiectasis.

Causes

1. Cystic fibrosis
2. Hypogammaglobulinemia
3. Kartagener syndrome in adults: Infection by *M. tuberculosis*, pneumonia, sinusitis.

In children the causes for bronchiectasis sicca are:
1. Foreign body obstruction of the bronchus
2. Following measles, a whooping cough.

Symptoms

1. Cough with copious expectoration in the morning
2. Hemoptysis
3. Breathlessness.

Signs

Finger clubbing.

Investigations

1. X-ray: Linear opacities at base as it is common in all the lower lobes of lungs.
2. Sputum culture must be done.

Complications

1. Lung abscess
2. Pleural effusion

3. Empyema
4. Brain abscess
5. Amyloidosis

Treatment

1. Removal of secretions by postural drainage
2. Antibiotics

Surgery

Segmentectomy or lobectomy.

Pulmonary rehabilitation program: Same as of pneumothorax (Refer page 131).

BRONCHOSTENOSIS

Definition

It is the chronic narrowing of the bronchus.

Site

Right main stem bronchus.

Clinical Features

Wheeze, stridor leads to lobar collapse or segmental collapse and lobar hyperinflation.

Causes

1. **Congenital:** This is very rare and occurs secondary to inflammatory changes following improper frequent suctioning of the infant on ventilatory support. Lung distal to stenosis becomes chemically infected as emphysematous.
2. **Traumatic:** Partial bronchial tears may remain unnoticed during the initial examination but these tears may lead to fibrosis and stricture formation is seen in the distal part of the lung.
3. **Infectious:** The main causes are as follows:
   a. *Tuberculosis:* Chronic infection leads to progressive destruction of bronchus and when healing occurs it heals by fibrosis resulting in stricture.
   b. *Histoplasmosis:* It causes mediastinal or hilar lymphadenopathy. At times, it can lead to excessive fibrosis following

healing of primary lesion. This enhanced fibro-genetic response may cause stenosis of adjacent bronchi.
4. **Postsurgical or iatrogenic:** Following lobectomy or lung transplantation.
5. In small cell lung carcinoma the radiation induced bronchostenosis is seen following post-radiation treatment
6. Prolonged endotracheal intubation.

Diagnosis

a. Chest X-ray: Shows distal collapse
b. Bronchoscopy
c. CT scan of the chest

Treatment

1. **Congenital:** In congenital conditions the repeated bronchodilation is done using nebulizer medication and if required chest physical therapy is performed.
2. **Traumatic:** Depends on presence of distal infection or not:
   a. If no infection is present, resect the stricture or primary repair of bronchus is done.
   b. If infection is present then lung resection is done.
3. **Infection:** Surgical resection or reconstruction.
4. **Iatrogenic:**
   a. Lobectomy: Endoscopic shunt placements, pneumonectomy.
   b. Right main stem stenosis repeated dilution and endobronchial stunts are done.
   c. Left main stem stenosis, endobronchial stunts are done.

MASSIVE HEMOPTYSIS

Definition

The coughing up blood from lower respiratory tract or the coughing of about 100–600 mL of blood in 24 hours is called massive hemoptysis.

Pseudo-massive Hemoptysis

Coughing of blood from oral cavity or gastrointestinal tract.

Contents

Blood stained sputum and frank hemoptysis.

Causes

Pulmonary infection, mitral stenosis, left ventricular failure, tumors such as carcinoma, adenoma, endobronchial metastasis and pulmonary infraction, trauma.

Iatrogenic causes such as pulmonary contusion, transbronchial biopsy and transthoracic needle biopsy.

- **Hemorrhagic diathesis:** Purpura, leukemia, hemophilia;
- **Pulmonary hemorrhage:** Hemorrhagic fevers, good pastures syndrome, idiopathic pulmonary hemosiderosis, pulmonary vasculitis and Behcet's syndrome.
- **Vascular abnormalities:** A-V malformations, hereditary hemorrhagic telangiectasia, anticoagulant use, idiopathic, inflammatory conditions such as acute bronchitis, pulmonary infarction like a presence of a foreign body.

Investigations

1. **Sputum:** Malignant and tuberculous bacilli
2. **X-ray:** Pulmonary TB
3. **Blood:** RBC count
4. **Larynx:** For ulceration
5. **Bronchoscopy:** Exclude foreign body and malignant growth
6. **Bronchography:** Bronchiectasis
7. **Needle aspiration biopsy:** Intrapulmonary lesions
8. **Pulmonary angiography:** Anomalies of vascular structure
9. **CT scan:** Pulmonary infarction and lung carcinoma
10. **Thoracotomy:** If all of the above fails

Indications

Indications of hemoptysis are problems with lung blood vessels, infections and cancer.

Treatment

The treatment is divided into four sections:
1. **Identifying the bleeding site:** The patient should get adequate oxygenation if lung bleeding is the primary source of bleeding; bleeding site can be lung if there is a history of lung disease. Bleeding in lung can be found by auscultation. There is a gurgling sound. Patient can also feel abnormal sensation at the bleeding site.

2. **Positioning of the patient:** Patient has to be positioned on dependent side. If there is right lung bleeding, the patient should be placed on the right side and vice versa so the nonbleeding lung can be protected. If there is spillage of blood, it prevents gas exchange by blocking the airway with clot or alveoli with blood.
3. **Establish a patent airway/adequate gas exchange:** The patient has symptoms like shortness of breath, hemodynamic instability, poor gas exchange, or ongoing hemoptysis.
4. **Establish adequate cardiovascular function:** The following is done for the patients with less cardiopulmonary reserve. Mechanical ventilation or intubation is performed when there is right lung bleeding and also to protect the left lung from spilling the blood from right lung. So size 8 endotracheal tube is used for the intubation.

SUPPURATIVE LESIONS OF THE LUNG

1. Bronchiectasis
2. Lung abscess
3. Bronchopneumonia
4. Aspergillosis

Bronchiectasis

Definition

The bronchiectasis is the destructive lung disease characterized by the chronic dilatation of the bronchi associated with persistent variable inflammatory process in the lungs.

Causes

1. Infection
2. Inflammation
3. Bronchial obstruction
4. Pulmonary fibrosis

Signs

1. Bronchitis
2. Fibrosis
3. Consolidation
4. Cavitation
5. Collapse

Symptoms

1. Bronchiectasis sicca
2. Hemorrhage
3. Cough
4. Obstruction by foreign body

Complications

1. Pulmonary such as pneumonia, lung abscess and hemoptysis
2. Pleural: Pleural effusion, empyema
3. Pericarditis
4. Sinusitis
5. Cerebral abscess

Investigations

1. Sputum
2. X-ray
3. Lung function tests

Treatment

Medical
Tetracycline.

Physiotherapy
Physical therapy treatment: The treatment should be performed twice a day. Once in the morning for 15 to 20 min because the secretions accumulate during night. So the techniques performed are deep breathing exercises, coughing, postural drainage techniques and position of the patient depends on the lobe to be drained and using clapping and percussion techniques during postural drainage. The same is performed in the evening too.

Pulmonary rehabilitation program: Same as of pneumothorax (Refer page 131).

Chemotherapy
Chemotherapy is required according to the stage of the disease. For mild conditions intermittent therapy is required and for severe cases continuous therapy is required.

Surgical treatment
Surgical resection: One segment or lobe is resected and in cases of hemoptysis; excision of the bronchial artery and embolization is done.

Contraindications

1. Old age
2. Poor cardiorespiratory function
3. Bilateral extensive disease (only 7-8 segments must be removed)

Lung Abscess

Definition

The localized formation of pus surrounded by a fibrous capsule within the lung tissue is called lung abscess.

Etiology

This is secondary to bronchial carcinoma.

Age

Over 40 years.

Causes

1. Inhalation of a foreign body.
2. Bacteria entering through the air passage because of bronchopneumonia.
3. Knife stab or bullet caused wound; the bacteria enters through the open chest wall.
4. Blood stream.
5. Secondary to bronchial carcinoma and abscess forms where secretion accumulates distal to the tumor.

Clinical Features

1. Fever
2. Dyspnea
3. Malaise
4. Pain
5. Cough which is irritable, unproductive. Initially productive of foul smelling sputum with bad taste in the mouth
6. Hemoptysis
7. Halitosis

Pathology

Inflammation of the lung tissue and suppuration occurs by invading organisms. Necrosis occurs in the center of the lung tissue with liquefaction and suppuration. The area becomes distended and fibroblasts lay down fibrous tissue around the area. Capsule contracts, abscess bursts resulting in the foul smelling sputum. Healing occurs with the formation of a fibrous scar.

Complications

1. Empyema.
2. Bronchiectasis: If the drainage spills into adjacent into lung tissue causes bronchiectasis.
3. Septicemia: Toxins from the pus can be absorbed into the blood stream.

Diagnosis

Radiograph: Shows fluid level.

Treatment

Antibiotics for 6 weeks.

Prognosis

The patient recovers with appropriate treatment.

Bronchopneumonia

Definition

It is a patchy and scattered lung condition in the lower lobes.

Etiology

Age: First 2 years and elderly.

Predisposing Factors

1. Weak and marasmic children
2. Rickets and infective fevers like measles and whooping cough

Onset

The patient may feel weak in the early stages.

Signs

1. Dullness to percussion
2. Fine crackles

Symptoms

1. Fever
2. Vomiting
3. Convulsions
4. Inflammation of nasal, pharyngeal or tracheobronchial passages
5. Dyspnea
6. Cough
7. Cyanosis
8. Gastrointestinal symptoms in infants such as vomiting, diarrhea
9. Nervous symptoms such as convulsions and meningitis

Treatment

1. Diet
2. Sedatives for distressing and restless patient
3. Antibiotics such as penicillin
4. Bronchodilators to reduce bronchospasm
5. Cyanosis: Humidified oxygen with blood gas monitoring
6. Metabolic acidosis: $NaHCO_3$
7. Fever: Paracetamol
8. Fluids: If the respiratory rate is >60/min
9. Other measures: Increase in the lung volume, improve gas exchange and clear secretions

Aspergillosis

Definition

Aspergillosis is a suppurative lesion of the lung that occurs due to filamentous fungi.

Causes

The agriculture workers are at specific risk.

Pathology

The fungus may infect a lung that is previously damaged by a tuberculous cavity, unsclerosed pneumonia, pulmonary pneumonia, and bronchiectasis.

Types

1. Allergic bronchopulmonary aspergillosis type-I
2. Aspergilloma—mycetoma type-II
3. Invasive aspergillosis type-III

Clinical Features

Type-I
1. Individuals will be hypersensitive, high titers of IgE, IgG
2. Inflammation of medium size bronchi
3. In asthma patients worsening of the air flow obstruction and cough
4. Proximal bronchiectasis.

Type-II
1. Cavities with TB will become colonized by *Aspergillus fumigatus*. A ball like fungal mass mixed with inflammatory debris and blood forms in the cavity which becomes lined with highly vascular granulation tissue.
2. Hemoptysis
3. Severe bleeding

Type-III
1. Severe neutropenia
2. T-lymphocyte deficient
3. Acute or subacute illness
4. Fever
5. Local cavitary pneumonia or disseminated pneumonia

Treatment

Type-I
Prednisolone 20–30 mg/day for 4–6 weeks, followed by maintenance with inhaled corticosteroids.

Type-II
Lobectomy for severe hemoptysis.

Type-III
Amphoterin.

CARCINOMA OF LUNG

Etiology

1. Smoking: Chances of active smokers are 85% and passive smokers are 3%.
2. Environmental risk factors from radon, asbestos, chromium, silica, nickel, and arsenic.
3. Pre-existing lung disease: COPD, pulmonary fibrosis.

Clinical Features

1. Cough
2. Hemoptysis
3. Dyspnea
4. Chest pain
5. Wheeze
6. **Nerves affected:**
    a. Phrenic nerve causes cough and paresis of diaphragm
    b. Recurrent laryngeal nerve causes hoarseness of voice
    c. Cervical sympathetic: Horner's syndrome
    d. Vagus nerve: Gastric symptoms
    e. Brachial plexus: Lower part will be involved
    f. Esophagus: Dysphagia
7. **Blood vessels:** Arteries and veins.
    a. *Superior vena cavae:* Venous engorgement of head and neck
    b. *Azygos vein:* Dilatation of superficial veins on thorax
    c. *Thoracic outlet:* Effusion
    d. *Axillary vessels:* Loss of peripheral pulses and edema of arm
8. **Erosion of rib:** Local pain and bony tenderness
9. Invasion of heart and pericardium
10. Bony metastasis in ribs and vertebrae
11. Hepatic metastasis
12. Suprarenal metastasis results in Addison's disease
13. **Endocrine abnormalities:**
    a. Cushing syndrome
    b. Hyponatremia
    c. Hypercalcemia
    d. Hypoglycemia
    e. Hyperthyroidism
    f. Gynecomastia
14. **Skeletal:**
    a. Finger clubbing with painful swelling of the wrists, ankles
    b. The periosteal new bone formation occurs on tibia, fibula, radius, and ulna
15. **Skin:** Eczematoid, bullous rashes
16. **Neurological:**
    a. Encephalopathy with dementia
    b. Cerebellar damage

c. Cerebellar degenerating syndrome
   d. Extrapyramidal syndrome
   e. Myelopathy
   f. Neuropathy
   g. Myasthenic syndrome
   h. Motor neuron disease
17. **Muscular:**
   a. Polymyositis
   b. Dermatomyositis
18. **Vascular:**
   a. Thrombophlebitis migrans
   b. Nonbacterial endocarditis
19. **Hematological:**
   a. Hemolytic anemia
   b. Thrombocytopenia
   c. Red cell aplasia

Diagnosis

1. History and physical examination.
2. Sputum cytology.
3. **Chest X-ray:** Localize the primary lesion. This can be central or peripheral.
4. **Computed tomography:** Assessing the primary tumor.
5. **Magnetic resonance imaging:** Assessing tumor, invasion into the spinal cord, vertebral bodies, and brachial plexus.
6. **Bronchoscopy:** This is one by either rigid or flexible bronchoscope. This allows the visualization up to third order bronchus and plays an essential role in the diagnosis, staging and treatment of lung cancer.
7. **Percutaneous needle biopsy:** Fluoroscopic or CT-guided needle biopsy successfully diagnoses lung cancer with ≥85–90% of accuracy.

Management

Radiotherapy

Indications
1. Early stage of disease
2. Refuse surgery
3. Medically unfit for surgery

Effects and uses
1. Hemoptysis, cough, chest-pain are reduced.
2. Temporarily relieve superior vena cava obstruction.
3. Compression of the esophagus or major bronchus is relieved.

Preoperative radiotherapy
1. For pancoast tumors
2. Prior to surgical resection

Postoperative radiotherapy
The postoperative radiotherapy is performed according to the patient and the condition based on the assessment.

Palliative radiotherapy
Palliative radiotherapy provides symptomatic relief for malignant bronchial obstruction and endobronchial tumor hemoptysis.

Brachytherapy
This involves the treatment of a tumor by direct application of radioactive sources that requires delivery of a localized high dose of radiotherapy. The radioactive source may be placed interstitially (directly into the tumor) or intracavitary (within the airway using a bronchoscopically placed after loading catheter).

Complications
1. Esophagitis
2. Pneumonitis
3. Pericarditis
4. Myelitis

Chemotherapy

Chemotherapy is one of the important therapies for overall management of lung cancer.

Chemotherapeutic agents
Cisplatin, mitomycin C, vindesine, vinblastine and ifosfamide.

Combination Therapy

The combination therapy improves quality of life.

Postoperative chemotherapy
1. Cisplatin and vinorelbine.
2. Taxol and carboplatin are administered.

Induction chemotherapy
It is a type of chemotherapy performed only when there is intact blood supply to the tumor so there is better delivery of chemotherapeutic agents before surgery and during radiotherapy.

Concurrent chemoradiotherapy
The chemoradiotherapy offers systemic and local control.

Surgical Treatment

This is the most effective treatment for early stages because primary tumor can be resected completely perioperative risk is low.

Preoperative evaluation must be one
1. Cardiovascular assessment
2. Pulmonary assessment
3. Prediction of postoperative morbidity with regard to
   a. Cardiovascular disease
   b. Pulmonary disease
   c. Age
   d. General medical condition
   e. Nutritional status
   f. Diabetes
   g. Immunosuppression
   h. Tumor stage
   i. Extent of resection
   j. Psychological factors

Preoperative preparation
1. Improve cardiopulmonary function
2. Cessation of smoking
3. Treatment of bronchospasm with bronchodilators and steroids
4. Reduction of the pulmonary secretions by chest physiotherapy and antibiotics
5. Correction of the anemia
6. Rehydration of the nutritional support
7. Correction of specific disorders such as congestive cardiac failure and cardiac dysrhythmias

Surgical principles
A complete resection of the primary tumor and its intrapulmonary lymphatics is essential. This is achieved by anatomic resection such as lobectomy or pneumonectomy, segmentectomy.

Stages I and II

Lobectomy, bilobectomy, and pneumonectomy are the surgical treatment of choice. Lesser resections such as wedge, segmentectomy should be reserved for high-risk patients who cannot tolerate lobectomy.

Surgical options

1. **Wedge or segmental resection:** The indications such as peripheral lung tumors in patient with poor pulmonary reserve. Recurrent rate is higher and survival is reduced.
2. **Lobectomy or bilobectomy:** This is a complete resection of hilar lymph nodes draining the primary tumor and allows preservation of the lung function.
3. **Pneumonectomy:** This accounts for 20% of all lung resection.
4. **Main stem bronchus or main pulmonary artery:** This procedure causes loss of lung parenchyma with significant chronic respiratory impairment.

THORACIC SURGERY

Thoracic Incisions

The thoracic incisions depends on the operation to be performed as well as the underlying pathology. Before planning the surgery, the correlation with the preoperative radiographic imaging is essential. The most common incisions used in the thoracic surgery includes are as follows:
1. Anterolateral thoracotomy
2. Posterolateral thoracotomy
3. Median sternotomy
   The knowledge of the thoracic cage and musculature is necessary.

Thoracic Cage

The thoracic cage consists of sternum anteriorly, the thoracic vertebrae posteriorly, and 12 pairs of the thoracic ribs connecting the both.

Thoracic Cage Musculature

This consists of two layers of muscles. They are as follows:
1. The intrinsic musculature consists of three intercostal muscle layers which are used for the respiration and protection.

2. The extrinsic muscles of respiration helps for stabilization of the thoracic cage and also acts as accessory muscles of respiration. The muscles are pectoralis major, serratus anterior, latissimus dorsi and sternocleidomastoid muscles.

Thoracotomy

A thoracotomy is a thoracic cavity incision for lungs, bronchi, and heart.

This is of two types:
1. **Lateral thoracotomy:** This is of two types. They are as follows:
   a. Anterolateral thoracotomy
   b. Posterolateral thoracotomy
2. **Anterior thoracotomy:** This is of two types. They are as follows:
   a. Transverse thoracotomy
   b. Vertical thoracotomy

Lateral Incisions

Anterolateral Thoracotomy

The incision is close to midline, in front follows along the line of a rib below the breast to the posterior axillary line. The muscles involved are pectoralis major, pectoralis minor, serratus anterior, internal intercostal, and external intercostal.

Indications
1. Pleurectomy
2. Mitral valvotomy
3. Open lung biopsy
4. Mobilization of the thoracic esophagus for resection
5. Lung resection

Operative technique
The patient is placed in the supine position with a roll placed vertically under the back and pelvis to raise the operated side by 45°. The ipsilateral arm is placed at the side. The incision is in the fourth or fifth intercostal space. The musculature is divided and a portion of the costal cartilage may be removed for extra exposure.

Advantages
1. Few muscles are divided.

Disadvantages
1. Limited exposure
2. Painful exposure

3. Higher incidence of the lung herniation since the intercostal space is more difficult to close

Posterolateral Thoracotomy

The incision is at vertebral border of the scapula and the line of a rib such as 5, 6, 7, or 8 to the anterior angle or costal margin. The muscles involved are trapezius, latissimus dorsi and rhomboids major, serratus anterior, intercostal, and erector spinae. To assess to the thorax if required, a rib may be removed or some are retracted.

Indications
1. Lung operation
2. Unilateral lung resection
3. Esophageal surgery
4. Chest-wall tumor resection
5. Unilateral lung volume reduction surgery/bullectomy
6. Tumors of the posterior mediastinum

Technique
The patient is placed in the lateral decubitus position with careful attention to padding pressure points such as the elbows and knees, and the lateral position is maintained by the adhesive tape, sandbags, or a vacuum bean bag. The incision is done measuring two finger width below the tip of the scapula along the line of the ribs and can be extended posteriorly in a vertical direction between the scapula and the spine. Some muscles incised others are retracted according to the requirement. Fifth space is selected for the lung resections.

Advantages
1. Good access to all regions of the thoracic cavity
2. Uncommon postoperative infections

Disadvantages
Increased postoperative pain secondary to muscle transection or displacement of the ribs.

Median Sternotomy

This is the subdivision of anterior thoracotomy incision and also called the vertical anterior thoracotomy.

Indications
1. Open heart surgery
2. Mediastinal tumor resection

3. Bilateral lung volume reduction surgery/bullectomy
4. Resection of the multiple pulmonary lesions
5. Transpericardial access to trachea/bronchus
6. Trauma

Technique
The patient is placed in the supine position with a roll placed under the shoulders. A vertical incision is made from the sternal notch to the xiphoid process or upper abdomen and the retrosternal space beneath the manubrium and the xiphoid process is mobilized. Pectoral fascia is incised in the midline and the sternum is split in the midline and mediastinal connective tissue is divided. The sternum is reapproximated using a tout stainless-steel wire and the pectoralis fascia is closed with a heavy absorbable suture.

Advantages
Decreased postoperative pain because the incision is stable and muscles are not involved leading to improvement of the respiratory function and mobilization.

Disadvantages
1. Osteomyelitis
2. Sternal dehiscence
3. Posterior thoracic cavity on the left side is difficult to access

POSTOPERATIVE COMPLICATIONS

Atelectasis

Definition
The incomplete expansion of the lung and collapse of the alveoli is called atelectasis.

Clinical Features
Low grade temperature and rales on respiration.

Treatment
Deep diaphragmatic breathing, postural drainage with percussion and vibration if secretions are present.

Cardiac Arrest

Definition
The cessation of the function of the heart is called cardiac arrest.

Clinical Features

Breathlessness, pulselessness, paleness and unresponsive.

Treatment

Cardiopulmonary resuscitation, immediate medical attention, no Trendelenburg position, segmental breathing, elevate the bed to 45–60° and deep breathing is encouraged.

Cardiac Dysrhythmia

Definition

The irregularity in the normal rhythm of the heart is called cardiac dysrhythmia.

Clinical Features

Irregular pulse.

Treatment

The patient performs modified deep breathing exercises.

Bed Position

Bed should be in flat position and no elevation required.

Cardiac Tamponade

Definition

The heart is compressed secondary to fluid collected in the sac surrounding the heart. There is drastic drop in the blood pressure secondary to pressure on the heart that prevents from filling it completely.

Clinical Features

Decrease in the cardiac output, blood pressure, increased heart rate, and shortness of the breath.

Treatment

This is an emergency situation and emergency treatment is required. A small tube or needle is taken and fluid is drained out.

Congestive Cardiac Failure

Definition

The effusion of the serous fluid in the interstitial tissues of the lungs.

Clinical Features

Shortness of breath, diaphoresis, peripheral edema.

Treatment

Modified postural drainage, avoid head-down position, relaxation exercises.

Empyema

Definition

The accumulation of the pus in the pleural cavity is called empyema.

Clinical Features

Fever, weight loss, malaise, decreased breath sounds, and dull percussion over area.

Treatment

Segmental breathing, deep diaphragmatic breathing, increased mobility.

Hemothorax

Definition

The presence of the blood in the pleural cavity. If this is seen with pneumothorax, it is called hemopneumothorax.

Clinical Features

Pain, dyspnea, hypertension, diaphoresis, and shortness of breath.

Treatment

When stabilized segmental breathing on the involved side.

Hypercapnia

Definition

The increase of the carbon dioxide in arterial blood.

Clinical Features

Mental status change is seen.

Treatment

Oxygen therapy.

Hypoxia

Definition

The low oxygen content in the body from hypoventilation, ventilation-perfusion ratio imbalance or underlying pulmonary disease is called hypoxia.

Clinical Features

Headache, mental fatigue, poor judgment and decreased breath sounds.

Treatment

Medical treatment and effective breathing.

Pleural Effusion

Definition

The presence of the fluid in the pleural space is called pleural effusion.

Clinical Features

Shortness of breath, pain, dyspnea, decrease breath sounds, tubercular breath sounds from one or two intercostal spaces above effusion.

Treatment

To increase mobility the deep breathing exercise and segmental breathing exercises are performed. To remove the expectorant postural drainage is performed depending on the lobe. If the patient had shortness of breath then postural drainage is contraindicated.

Pneumonia

Definition

The inflammation of the alveoli usually from the blood-borne organisms.

Clinical Features

Fever and rales, chills and tubercular breath sounds, dyspnea and dull percussion, and painful inhalation.

Treatment

Deep breathing and coughing, postural drainage, percussion, and vibration.

Pneumothorax

Definition

The presence of air in the pleural cavity is called pneumothorax.

Clinical Features

Shortness of breath, dyspnea, diaphoresis and absence of breath sounds over the upper lobe area.

Treatment

To increase chest mobility segmental breathing exercises are performed, postural drain to remove the secretions and chest tube is inserted for removal of air.

Postcardiotomy Syndrome

Definition

This condition is the combination of the pericarditis, pleurisy, pneumonitis, and the pleural effusion.

Clinical Features

Thoracic pain, dyspnea, and shortness of breath.

Treatment

Percussion is contraindicated because of the pleuritic pain, segmental breathing is given for pleural effusion.

Pulmonary Embolism

Definition

The obstruction of the pulmonary artery or one of its branches by a clot.

Clinical Features

1. **Acute:** Pain, shortness of breath, dyspnea, tachycardia
2. **Subacute:** Hemoptysis, pleural effusion, friction rub, and decreased breath sounds over the involved area.

Treatment

Deep breathing, segmental breathing, postural drainage if the patient is stable, increase mobility, anticoagulant therapy, percussion, and vibration after 6 days after therapy.

Respiratory Arrest

Definition

The cessation of the respiratory function is called respiratory arrest.

Clinical Features

Increased or no respiratory rate, hypoxia and diaphoresis.

Treatment

Immediate medical treatment and cardiopulmonary resuscitation.

Respiratory Distress

Definition

The noticeable difficulty in breathing is called respiratory distress.

Clinical Features

Increased respiratory rate, secretions in the lungs, diaphoresis, hypoxia and anxiety.

Treatment

Oxygen therapy, drug therapy, suction, intubation, and extubation.

Subcutaneous Emphysema

Definition

The collection of the air in the subcutaneous tissue is called subcutaneous emphysema.

Clinical Features

Swelling and crackles are heard on palpation.

Treatment

Deep breathing should be avoided with large air leak, percussion is contraindicated over the swollen area.

Cardiogenic Shock

Definition

The sudden diminution of the cardiac output is called cardiogenic shock.

Clinical Features

Cardiac damage decreases the cardiac output and makes the patient hypotensive.

Treatment

Medical and drug therapy.

Deep Vein Thrombosis

Definition

The coagulation or the clot of the blood that remains at the site of the origin is called DVT.

Clinical Features

When the thrombus gets detached it becomes embolus and if the embolus travels to either side of the lungs it causes pulmonary embolism.

Causes

Venous stasis, trauma, dehydration and increased platelet counts.

Prevention: Ankle pumps pre- and postoperatively about 10–15 every hour.

Treatment

Flexion of the hip and knee is contraindicated. If the leg shows thrombophlebitis, the excessive movement, rolling should be avoided till the required anticoagulant therapy is given for about 4–5 days.

Other Complications

Respiratory

1. Infection of the lungs tissue.
2. Collapse of the remaining lung.
3. Bronchopleural fistula: This occurs when the stump of the bronchus from which the lungs tissue has been removed breaks down.

4. Pain is the major factor in reducing the lung volume causes guarding spasm of the trunk muscles and inhibits breathing. The reduced volume causes closed airways and absorption of the gas.
5. Prolonged recumbence affects the amount of the distribution of ventilation and cause intrathoracic pooling of blood that displaces a proportion of air in the lung.
6. Nausea because of the certain drugs, which inhibit deep breathing.
7. Fatigue.
8. Anxiety causes diaphragmatic splinting, increases surgical risks, and prolongs hospitalization.
9. Depression if the surgery causes altered body image.
10. Empyema.
11. Local gangrene: Pyrexia and hemoptysis.

Circulatory Complications

1. Cardiac tamponade
2. Hemorrhage
3. Chest infection
4. Cardiac herniation
5. Cardiac failure
6. Myocardial infarction

Wound Complications

1. Infection
2. Failure to heal
3. Adhesion scar formation

Joint Stiffness

1. Shoulder and shoulder girdle
2. Thoracic spine
3. Costovertebral joint

Muscle Weakness

1. Latissimus dorsi
2. Serratus anterior
3. Leg muscles if excised

Postural Deformity

The tendency to protect the scar leads to the scoliosis and forward flexion.

Digestive Complications

Hiccups cause sharp pain at the wound site.

Renal Complications

1. Decreased urine output
2. Oliguria causes renal failure
3. Anuria causes urinary tract obstruction
4. Renal vascular obstruction or acute cortical necrosis

INCISIONS, INDICATIONS, CONTRAINDICATIONS, AND COMPLICATIONS

Segmentectomy

Definition

The segmentectomy also called segmental resection is the surgical removal of a portion of gland or organ, e.g., lungs—the removal of lung tissue from one of the lobes of lungs or bronchopulmonary segment, for the treatment of breast cancer—removal of tumor breast tissue and below the tumor the removal of lining of the chest muscles, for the treatment of liver cancer removal of portion of liver affected.

Complications

Bronchopleural fistula and empyema.

Lobectomy

It is surgical removal of the part of organ, e.g., for the treatment of lung cancer—removal of the lobe of the lung, hemithyroidectomy is removal of lobe of thyroid, anterior temporal lobectomy is removal of lobe of the brain.

Indications

1. Bronchiectasis
2. TB
3. Lung abscess
4. Carcinoma
5. Fungus infection
6. Congenital and early childhood conditions

Contraindications

Surgery is performed only if the tumor is localized, based on the size and type of the tumor is also considered. But if there is metastasis into two or more areas of the body the surgery is contraindicated.

Complications

1. Peripheral adhesions
2. Incomplete fissures
3. Bronchopleural fistula
4. Postlobectomy empyema
5. Chronic empyema
6. Decreased lung capacity so patient has to use inhalers.

Pneumonectomy

Definition

It is the removal of the entire lung.

Indication

Bronchogenic carcinoma in males, breast cancer in females.

Types

- **Simple pneumonectomy:** The surgery includes removal of only affected lung.
- **Extra-pleural pneumonectomy:** This surgery is done in malignant mesothelioma conditions where the affected lung, parietal pleura, part of diaphragm, pericardium of the affected side are removed and the replaced with GORE-TEX.

Complications

1. When the patient respiratory capacity is decreased. The incentive spirometer is used to improve breathing function and to maintain exercise capacity of the remaining lung
2. Cardiovascular instability
3. Empyema
4. Bronchopleural fistula
5. Damage to the phrenic nerve
6. Damage to the recurrent laryngeal nerve.

Pleuropneumonectomy

It is also a type of pneumonectomy and it is the removal of pleura and the entire lung.

Tracheostomy

Definition

This is a procedure performed either as an emergency procedure or as a planned operation.

Indications

1. Upper airway obstruction
2. Tracheobronchial outlet
3. Airway assess for mechanical ventilation
4. Elimination of the dead space

Procedure

The patient in supine position with neck hyperextended and a transverse skin incision is made below the cricoid. Thyroid isthmus is retracted superiorly or inferiorly. A vertical incision of the second and third tracheal rings is used. A tracheostomy tube of appropriate size is inserted with the obturator in place and the cuff deflated. Tracheostomy tube is in place and the cuff deflated, the obturator is removed and a suction catheter is introduced through the tube. Free passage into the lower airway and the aspiration of tracheal secretions confirms proper placement. Cuff is inflated and the inner cannula placed prior to ventilation. The tube is sutured to the skin and a tracheostomy tape is tied around the neck to prevent dislodgement in the cavity during postoperative period.

Complication

1. **Intraoperative:**
   a. Bleeding
   b. Pneumothorax
   c. Hypoxia leading to cardiorespiratory arrest (misplacement of the tracheostomy tube into the pretracheal space)
2. **Postoperative:**
   a. Bleeding
   b. Wound infection
   c. Tube obstruction or displacement
   d. Swallowing difficulty

e. Tracheostenosis
f. Tracheoesophageal fistula
g. Tracheoinnominate artery fistula
h. Tracheocutaneous fistula

Postoperative Management

Postoperative care of a thoracic surgical patient begins in the operating room. A catheter is positioned in the radial artery for monitoring arterial blood pressure and blood gas analysis. Oxygen saturation is monitored and end tidal carbon dioxide mass spectrometry are used to monitor pulmonary function. Large central venous line is placed for intravenous fluid administration and also monitoring the right heart pressure. If the patient has history of cardiac and pulmonary disease a catheter is placed in the pulmonary artery for monitoring pulmonary capillary wedge pressure.

After completion of the intrathoracic operation procedure, large pleural drainage tubes are inserted into the thorax for suction and drainage from several different areas within the pleural cavity.

The pleural space should not be drained routinely following pneumonectomy. Intrapleural pressure should be regulated approximately −4 to −10 cm of water to prevent shifting of the mediastinum. This is done by an intercostal catheter connected to a manometric system or a needle simply inserted through a skin into the pleural cavity after procedure is completed. Once the intended pressure in the supine lying is achieved, the tube or the needle is removed.

After pneumonectomy suction should not be applied to the chest tubes because mediastinum may shift. Following closure of the thoracic wound postoperative care is divided into:
1. Immediate management
2. Early management
3. Late management

Immediate management
The immediate postoperative care is also performed in the operating room and the principal consideration is
- Protection of the wound
- Connection of the pleural drainage tubes to an underwater seal
- Maintenance of the adequate airway
- Transportation of the patient.

Protection of the wound: A light dressing is applied to the wound supported by elastic adhesive tape. The adjacent skin is first rescrubbed with an antiseptic agent followed by an application of tincture of benzoin. When allowed to dry, makes a sticky surface to which the elastic adhesive easily adheres without undue skin traction. This type of dressing avoids restriction of motion in the thoracic cage and allows coughing and deep breathing in the immediate postoperative period and this is removed next day after operation exposing the closed incision to the air.

Connection of the pleural drainage tubes to an underwater seal: Classical three bottle suction system is used. The first bottle is for collection and measurement of fluid drained from the chest. Aspiration of air back into the pleural space is prevented by an underwater seal in the second bottle. The negative intrapleural pressure is maintained by the third bottle which has a water column for regulating the amount of suction applied to the pleural space.

Maintenance of the adequate airway: Prolonged endotracheal intubation and mechanical ventilation is because of central nervous system (CNS) depression due to anesthetic agents, hypoxemia, possibility of continuing bleeding, inadequacy of cardiac performance.

Transportation of the patient: Oxygen administration by a facemask if the patient is extubated. If patient cannot be extubated, using an anesthetic bag and a portable oxygen delivery system must assist ventilation. Chest tubes should not be clamped during transport, if assisted ventilation is required, connect to an underwater seal.

Complications:
1. Tension pneumothorax
2. Cardiopulmonary collapse

Early management
Following arrival of the patient in the recovery room or intensive care unit, the arterial blood pressure, electrocardiogram, and oxygen saturation should be monitored continuously. This helps in immediate recognition of the problems. Heart and the respiratory rate should be recorded every 15 minutes until the patient is stable. Urinary output, chest drainage tubes, central venous pressure, and temperature are measured hourly. Body weight is recorded daily. Chest roentgenograms are the X-ray findings of the internal structures of lungs and heart. The report is taken every morning and every evening until the day when the chest tube is removed.

Pulmonary care: The patients with thoracic operations have abnormal function due to chronic obstructive lung disease. Postoperative pulmonary complications are reduced by chest PT, aerosolized bronchodilators, mist, hydration, antibiotics, and the avoidance of bronchial irritants.

Pleural space: Pleural drainage tubes must remain patent and frequently examined. The tube should be irrigated with 30 mL of sterile saline, milked throughout their length at frequent intervals to prevent clotted blood from occluding them. The amount of pleural drainage should be recorded at hourly intervals. Blood loss should be replaced by blood administration intravenously.

Medications: Following operation intermittent epidural administration of either local anesthetic such as morphine relieves pain, improves pulmonary function, and allows early ambulation.

Fluids and electrolyte: Intravenous fluid therapy consists of the administration of daily maintenance fluid plus fluid replacement of any losses. Administration of 1,000 mL of 5% dextrose and 0.2% NaCl per square meter of body surface area during the first 24 postoperative hours and 1,500 mL/m^2 for each subsequent 24-hour period is adequate to maintain fluid balance.

Gastric distention: Mechanical ventilation by mask or mouthpiece frequently forces air and anesthetic gases into the stomach. Nasogastric tube is passed into stomach to evacuate the gases and important after a right pneumonectomy where a distended stomach may interfere with movement of the left hemi diaphragm.

Late management

The problem of bronchial secretions reduces and coughing is no longer painful. The wound support is not required and dressing can be removed. The wound can be covered with a light gauze dressing or not required. If the wound is left open, care must be taken to avoid its irritation by rubbing against bedsheets, e.g., posterior thoracotomy wound, so frequent change of position and placement of the patient on a sheep skin cover is done. The patient should be up and out of bed.

Prolonged sitting especially with legs crossed should be avoided to prevent venous stasis. The patient should be encouraged to eat his meals sitting on a chair. By the third postoperative day, the patient should be on a general diet. The patient should be encouraged to take frequent warm showers after the drainage tubes are removed. Gentle bathing of the wound has a mild analgesic effect and provides relaxation.

Skin stitches may be removed on the 7th or 8th postoperative day. The use of absorbable subcuticular sutures greatly facilitates wound care postoperatively.

The medication should be stable and the patient should not have any complications for the patients, should be ambulatory and able to care for themselves, who are ready for hospital dismissal. An exercise program should be outlined that will prepare these patients for resumption of normal life activity and return them to their previous occupation without producing excessive fatigue or undue stress upon the operative wounds. Strenuous physical activity or lifting objects heavier than 10 lb is prohibited for 6 weeks. Patients are encouraged to walk or perform light exercise immediately upon discharge.

Oral narcotic analgesics are usually required at discharge and reduce after 1 month long-term pain occurs in about 1% of patients and referred to as post-thoracotomy pain syndrome. It is usually from intercostal nerve irritation and is effectively treated by local injection; TENS is helpful.

VENTILATORS

Definition

Ventilators are the devices used for artificial ventilation.

Indications

1. Respiratory failure
2. Crush injuries of the chest, severe scoliosis, major surgery
3. Muscular cases such as tetanus, myasthenia gravis, and muscular dystrophy
4. Pulmonary: Acute respiratory distress syndrome, chronic obstructive pulmonary disease, bronchial asthma, and drowning
5. CNS: Drugs, overdose of morphine, poising, epilepsy, cerebrovascular accident, and poliomyelitis

Types of Ventilators

1. **Negative pressure**: The whole body below neck is kept in a large negative tank and a negative pressure is set in tank which induces pressure.
2. **Positive pressure:** Air is sent into the lungs with pressure more than atmospheric pressure, i.e., supra-atmospheric pressure is set up and air is driven through trachea.
3. **High frequency positive**: This is of two types:
   a. Jet high frequency positive: 350 breathes/min
   b. Oscillator high frequency positive: 1,300 breathes/min

Modes of Ventilation

This is two types. They are as follows:
1. Full ventilatory support
2. Partial ventilatory support

The following explained below will provide full ventilator support and partial ventilator supply.
1. **Controlled mandatory ventilator:** This is the fixed ventilation for definite time intervals, no provision for spontaneous ventilatory effort, limited to intraoperative, and immediate postoperative ventilation.
2. **Assist control mode:** This acts like a controlled mandatory ventilator and when the patient takes a spontaneous breathe, the ventilator is triggered to reach a preset level of ventilation.
3. **Intermittent mandatory ventilator (IMV) and synchronized IMV (SIMV):** In IMV, the patient are free to breathe spontaneously between set ventilator breaths. Mandatory breathes may be synchronized with the patients spontaneous efforts.
   Advantages:
   a. Better gas distribution
   b. Lower mean airway pressure
   c. Less hemodynamic disturbance
   d. Less sedation is required
   e. Weaning is easier
4. **Pressure support ventilator:** A preset inspiratory pressure is added to the ventilator circuit during inspiration in spontaneously breathing patients.
5. **Controlled mechanical ventilator:** Tidal volume and the respiratory rate are set in machine.
6. **Assisted mechanical ventilator:** Tidal volume is set and useful in weaning.
7. **Assisted controlled ventilator:** The tidal volume is set and the patient is allowed to respire on their own.
8. **Intermittent mandatory ventilator:** The patient breathes on their own and in between breath rate is calculated.
9. **Synchronized mandatory ventilator:** When patient makes effort the machine itself calculates the requirement.
10. **Pressure ratio mandatory ventilator:** The ventilator sets the pressure in during the inspiration and sent to the machine.
11. **Inverse ratio ventilator:** Normal inspiration-expiration ratio is 1:1.5–1:2. The inspiration time is increased. This reading is useful for acute respiratory distress syndrome.

12. **Independent lung ventilator:** Bifid endotracheal tubes are used in patient when one side of lung is affected more than other.

Setting Up the Ventilator

1. Ensure the airway is secure
2. Ensure adequate sedation, opioids and muscle relaxants
3. Tidal volume: Normal (10 mL/kg body weight)
4. Respiratory rate: 14–16/min
5. Fraction of inspired oxygen: It is the amount of oxygen inspired in fraction of air. So medically ill patients who has difficulty in breathing are provided with 100% of oxygen air.

Factors to be Observed in Case of Ventilation

1. Vital signs such as blood pressure, heart rate
2. Consciousness of patient
3. Secretion should be removed periodically
4. Checks alarm function of the ventilator
5. Oxygen saturation in the blood

Classification of Ventilator on Phases

1. **Inspiratory phase:** This phase includes the following generators:
   a. *Pressure generators:* Exposes the lung to a pressure
   b. *Flow generators:* Exposes the lung to the low of gas
2. **Cycling or change over to expiration:** This phase includes the following:
   a. *Pressure-cycled ventilator:* The oxygen is allowed to flow into the lungs until airway pressure limit is reached then the valve opens for exhalation. The types of pressure cycled ventilators are Bird ventilator, Blease ventilator, Aarlow ventilator and Cyclator ventilator.
   b. *Volume-cycled ventilator:* The oxygen flows to the patient's lungs until the preset volume is delivered. The volume varies with airway resistant changes and lung compliance. The types of volume cycled ventilator are Bear ventilator, Bennect ventilator, Monaghan ventilator, Brompton ventilator.
   c. *Time-cycled:* The mechanical ventilator switches from inspiration to expiration and depends on inspiration-expiration ratio, respiratory rate and inspiratory time. The types of timed cycled ventilator are Servo ventilator, Clape ventilator, Phillips ventilator and Engstrom ventilator.

3. **Expiratory phase**: Positive end expiratory pressure (PEEP) and negative end expiratory pressure (NEEP) allow expiratory restriction or choice to be used so that expiration is slowed. PEEP is a positive pressure and NEEP is a negative pressure.
4. **Cycling to inspiration**: This phase sets function independently without patient so called controlled ventilation.
   a. *Intermittent mandatory ventilation (IMV)*: The patient breathes spontaneously in between machine breaths. Machine breaths are delivered at set frequency, inspiratory flow rate and tidal volume.
   b. *Mandatory minute volume (MMV)*: This gives the patient slight assistance to her own spontaneous efforts.
   c. *Continuous positive airway pressure (CPAP)*: This continuous positive airway pressure is recommended for patients with mild to moderate acute respiratory insufficiency, median sternotomy and coronary artery bypass graft (CABG). This increases functional residual capacity and improves oxygenation.

Complications

1. Due to endotracheal tube
2. Barotrauma increases pressure—surgical emphysema, pneumothorax
3. Fluid retention
4. Stress ulcers—gastric or duodenal

PREOPERATIVE ASSESSMENT AND MANAGEMENT OF A PATIENT POSTED FOR THORACOTOMY

The preoperative preparation of the patient includes the following measures:

Preoperative Assessment

1. **Chart review**: The chest should be reviewed with special attention to tests and studies related to the surgery to be done.
2. **Patient interview**: The patient's interview can contribute useful information regarding a patient.
   a. Family history
   b. Occupation
   c. Habits such as smoking, use of alcohol
   d. Pulmonary symptom, frequency and pattern

e. Functional activities must be assessed for determination of appropriate postoperative goals for the patients
3. **Physical assessment:**
   a. *Observation:*
      i. Color
      ii. Breathing pattern: Rate, amplitude, rhythm
      iii. Mental state
      iv. Posture
      v. Body build
      vi. Supportive equipment
      vii. Secretion
      viii. Patient ability to move
      ix. Skin
      x. Scars
   b. *Palpation:* Bilateral palpation of the thorax allows comparison of the symmetry of the following physical signs
      i. Equality of thoracic movement: Equality of thoracic movement is based on the lateral coastal expansion, apical expansion, posterior thoracic basal expansion and diaphragmatic excursion
      ii. Vocal fremitus
   c. *Auscultation and percussion:* This is important to establish a baseline assessment of chest sound, adventitious breath sounds are noticed, preoperatively treatment to improve pulmonary status before surgery.
   d. *Range of motion:* The preoperative range of motion is necessary to observe preoperative range of motion and to determine goals of postoperative mobility, emphasis should be given to joints that will be affected by incised musculature.

Preoperative Condition

The preoperative course decreases the following:
1. The patient's length of stay from surgery to discharge
2. The number of postoperative complications
3. The number of PT treatment required postoperatively
4. The preoperative session is the session prior to the surgery where it helps the patient and physical therapist. The interaction is to motivate and prepare the patient for the surgery and also postoperative complications to be expected and importance of postoperative physical therapy session.

Preoperative Session

Major points to be covered during preoperative session are:

Rationale for Treatment

Explanation about the treatment in detail which includes the following points:
1. Effect of bed rest
2. Immobility on pulmonary status
3. Respiratory depression from anesthesia
4. Appropriate lung response to the surgeries
5. All the above will decrease aeration and increase mucous production.

Surgical Procedure

A brief description of the surgical procedure is offered:
1. Incision placement
2. Length of surgery
3. Details depend on the patient's level of understanding

Monitoring and Supportive Devices

Patient is explained about the monitoring and supportive devices:
1. Foley catheter: To collect urine output and monitor kidney function
2. Chest tubes to drain the thoracic cavity of any accumulation of air or fluid
3. Intravenous tubes to maintain nutrition and hydration
4. Cardiac monitor and electrodes to follow cardiac status
5. Arterial line to provide an access for arterial blood samples or blood gas analysis and for injection of medication
6. Left arterial pressure line to measure cardiac function
7. Endotracheal tube to provide an artificial airway for respiratory assistance by a ventilator
8. Nasogastric tube to drain gastric secretion

PULMONARY REHABILITATION

The pulmonary rehabilitation is a multidisciplinary program of a patient with acute and chronic respiratory diseases that are designed to increase the overall quality of life of the patient. Pulmonary rehabilitation is for the patients who are diagnosed with respiratory ailments or pulmonary diseases.

Indications

1. Chronic respiratory failure
2. COPD such as asthma, bronchitis, bronchiectasis, cystic fibrosis
3. Reduced capacity to perform dailylife activities
4. Dyspnea
5. Surgical intervention

Contraindications

1. Pulmonary hypertension
2. Ischemic heart disease
3. Liver dysfunction
4. Cancer
5. Renal failure

Uses

1. Pulmonary rehabilitation helps patient to understand the disease, treatment and rehabilitation plan, and progress
2. Pulmonary rehabilitation improves quality of life
3. Pulmonary rehabilitation decreases anxiety, depression secondary to lung condition
4. Pulmonary rehabilitation deals with weather precautions like not too cold or not too hot and care to be taken during weather changes
5. Pulmonary rehabilitation decreases hospital stay
6. Pulmonary rehabilitation helps in good understanding of medications use, side effects.

Phases of Pulmonary Rehabilitation

The pulmonary rehabilitation is divided into two phases
1. Preoperative pulmonary rehabilitation
2. Postoperative pulmonary rehabilitation

Preoperative Pulmonary Rehabilitation

The postoperative treatment is demonstrated with the patient rolling, positioning for bronchial drainage, percussion, vibration, splinting, coughing are practiced. This provides the patient the required treatment after surgery. The therapist can divide the treatment part into five areas. They are:

1. **Deep breathing**
   a. Improves alveolar ventilation which is very important.
   b. Prevents postoperative pulmonary complications.
   c. Breathing exercises are taught in semi-Fowler's position where abdominal muscles are slack.
   d. This position allows greater diaphragmatic excursion.
   e. This is emphasized as a modality for postoperative pulmonary hygiene.
   f. Depending upon the patient's capability, it is taught to the patient. For example, some patient can breathe effectively with their diaphragm so only encouragement is done to fully aerate their lungs. Some patient finds the technique difficult, so need additional care. This promotes relaxation and reduces anxiety.
2. **Rolling:** Rolling technique minimizes trunk movement and allows patient mobility. The patient is encouraged to flex at the hips and knees and roll with the shoulders and hips.
3. **Coughing:** Anesthesia and surgery causes decreased cough effectiveness. The cough with bronchial drainage, shaking percussion accelerates central and peripheral lung clearance.

   There are two stages of cough: (1) Full-raises secretion, (2) Deep diaphragmatic facilitates expectoration. Bigger is the breathe stronger will be cough. Patients are instructed to apply pressure over the incision by using pillows or their hands or it may cause pain near the incision area. The patient will be taught huffing. Huffing is an effective mode of secretion mobilization and may be used as an alternative in patient who has an ineffective cough.

   Huffing is an accomplished by forceful expiration through an open glottis. The patient is asked to say the word huff and attempt to elongate the letter H. Repetition of the maneuver stimulates spontaneous cough.
4. **Incentive spirometry:** It is an adjunct to breathing exercises that provides the patient with visual feedback of the volume of inspired air during a deep breathe. The patient is encouraged to practice deep inspiration every hour, chest PT session. Maximum inhalation with incentive spirometry inflates alveoli and decreases postoperative complications. Others are IPPB (intermittent positive pressure breathing) and PEEP.
5. **Ankle circles:** Use of ankle pump to minimize the incidence of phlebitis facilitates venous return.

   These preoperative sessions strengthen the patient therapist relationship. The patient feels confident meeting the therapist who will tract them through their hospital course.

Postoperative Pulmonary Rehabilitation

Please refer to Pulmonary Rehabilitation Management in this book.

S. No.	Aims of physical therapy	Plans of physical therapy
1.	To mobilization and removal of secretion	Active and passive techniques are used. Active technique where the patient performs by himself and passive techniques where physical therapist helps patient to perform the technique to remove secretions.
		Passive techniques are postural drainage, percussion, vibration and forced expiratory techniques like coughing and huffing *Active techniques:* ACBT (active cycle breathing techniques), thoracic expansion exercises, forced expiratory techniques like coughing and huffing
2.	To improve breathing efficiency	Breathing exercises like diaphragmatic breathing, segmental breathing, lateral costal breathing, glossopharyngeal breathing, and pulse lip breathing
3.	To teach postural awareness	Postural education and ergonomic training
4.	To strengthen the muscles	Strengthening exercises using Theraband and weights
5.	To teach energy conservation and reduce fatigue	Activity pacing and energy conservation techniques
6.	To reduce stress	Yoga and medication

The above mentioned techniques should be carefully performed as the patient is recovering from the surgery. Till surgical incision is healed it should always be protected. All these techniques to be performed as per patient's requirement and tolerance.

Postsurgical Physical Therapy Intervention

The priority is emphasizing on protection and healing of surgical incision. Utmost care should be taken during physical therapy session starting with patient education, positioning, activity tolerance.

ENDOTRACHEAL/ENDONASAL TUBES

Endotracheal Tube

The endotracheal tube is passed through the mouth or nose. It is used when the patient cannot maintain his/her own airway. The tube passed through mouth is called oral endotracheal tube and the tube passed through nose is called nasal endotracheal tube.

Oral Intubation

Patient has to be educated not to clamp using his or her teeth on the oral tube or it may lead to obstruct the airway.

Nasal Intubation

The nasal intubation overcomes the problem, but longer tube of smaller diameter has to be used. There is a risk of sinusitis as tube may block the nasal sinus.

Tracheostomy

It is an operation to create an opening or stoma into the trachea. The patient will be more comfortable. The patient will be on Trach, ventilator and oxygen in liters depending on the requirement and once the patient is stable. He or she will be weaned from the ventilator. Initially for short duration of 30 min and slowly progress to 24 hours under close monitoring of respiratory therapist and physical therapist treatment is done during the weaning period to know the patient activity tolerance and fatigue levels. If the patient is tolerating then the patient will be discharged from the ventilator and slowly Trach will be removed and patient is put on oxygen using nasal cannula.

Functions of Endotracheal or Tracheostomy Tube

1. To facilitate access to pulmonary secretion.
2. To prevent substances from the mouth entering and soiling the lungs.
3. To help to maintain positive pressure ventilation by preventing air from escaping around the tube.
4. To pass by an obstruction preventing ventilation. All endotracheal tube and tracheostomy tube decrease anatomical dead space by half size. Neonatal is 2.5 mm, adult is 0.5-11.0 mm. The silver tracheostomy tube is used in intermediate stage before finally closing the tracheostomy. It is an important feature for patients following laryngectomy. It has an inner tube that can be removed for cleaning. Some tubes have a value that allows the patient to speak.

Disadvantages

1. Increase danger of infection
2. Loss of humidification
3. Dry gases can be cause blockage of respiratory passage

Description of Endotracheal Tube

The tube is simple made up of plastic, has a right angle curve so that it fits over the tongue and pharynx. Airway vary in size, facilitates artificial ventilation.

Uses

1. The suffocation of the unconscious patient is prevented by the tongue falling backward.
2. Tube gives clear way for suction in unconscious and conscious patient.

Types

The endotracheal tubes used for the adult are plain type and cuffed type of endotracheal tubes for children and babies.

Endonasal Tubes

Definition

Endonasal tube is a tube to assist ventilation.

Material

Rubber, silicon, Teflon and PVC.

Variety

Two varieties are available. They are as follows:
1. Disposable
2. Autoclaved

Types

Two varieties, they are cuffed for adults and uncuffed for children.
- **Mode of intubation:** Nasal
- **Size:** Internal diameter
- **Adult male:** 9 mm
- **Adult female:** 6-8 mm
- **Children:** 4 mm (age till plus four)
- **Length:** Adult male and female—23-25 cm
- **Endotracheal tube:** For the children of age 2 years the length of endotracheal tube used are 12-15 cm in length.

Steps of Intubation

Endotracheal Tube

Anesthesia locally given with halothane 4%, suxamethonium muscle relaxin through right side of mouth through glottis below vocal cord with pressure of 25-30 mm of water.

Endonasal Tube

Passed through the floor of nose.

Uncuffed endotracheal tube: Pushed 3-4 cm behind the vocal cords, infants: <6 months: 2 cm, only neonates: 1 cm.

Complications of Endotracheal and Endonasal Tube

1. Injury to lips, teeth and oral cavity
2. Injury to nose, paranasal cavity
3. Eustachian tube infection leads to autitis, sinusitis, epistaxis, laryngitis, sore throat, tracheal stenosis. Kinking of tube, foreign body aspiration, tracheal tube obstruction can be kinking, biting, foreign body such as dried mucous, blood loss, pus, debris, granulation an defective tubes
4. Airway edema
5. Vocal cord dysfunction
6. Nasal damage
7. Dental or oropharyngeal complications

Nasogastric Tube Complications

1. Ulceration and necrosis of the nostrils
2. Esophageal reflex, esophagitis
3. Patient breaths with mouth instead of nose called mouth breathing
4. Interferes with ventilation and cough mechanism
5. Loss of fluid
6. Otitis media
7. Sinusitis
8. Traumatic laryngitis
9. Hoarseness of voice are seen.

Suction

Definition

Suction is a procedure that facilitates removal of bronchial secretion.

Suction Equipment

Suction apparatus such as electrical and portable, and foot pump.

Suction Tubing

Connections, catheters and suction trolley.

Suction Technique

Suction catheter introduced through nose and mouth.
Aim: To stimulate cough reflex.

Types

Nasopharyngeal, oropharyngeal, tube suction and minitracheostomy.

Minitracheostomy or Tracheal Suction

This is performed under local anesthesia. A narrow cannula is inserted surgically into the trachea then left in place for as many days as required. The patient is suctioned using 10 size U shape catheter through the aperture with the patient breathing normally throughout. The minitracheostomy preserves the function of the glottis so that coughing, speaking and eating are safe guarded, while spontaneous breathing a natural humidification are usual.

Uses

1. This is a simple procedure.
2. Bronchoscopy and intubation are not required.

Weaning

Definition

Weaning is the disconnection from the ventilator.

With few patients the weaning from the ventilator is easy. Example—younger age and present medical condition and severity of lung disease. Others with complications and lung disease severity need longer period of ventilator support and weaning may take longer duration. This period includes a trial of spontaneous breathing through the artificial airway during which the patient is assessed or extubation.

Weaning Difficulties

1. Damage of inspiratory muscles occurs due to lung disease.
2. Fear of suffocation.

Weaning is successful:
1. When maximum ventilatory reserve is present or airway is clear and baseline values or vital capacity, respiratory rate, inspiratory force and blood gases.
2. Optimal nutritional status, fluid, metabolic and cardiovascular status are present.
3. The maximum mobility, endurance are facilitated by practice in standing and walking.
4. Minimum sputum, maximum ability to cough are present.
5. Previous good night sleep is must.

Method

1. Explanation of the procedure is given to the patient.
2. Gradual reduction of ventilatory support can be achieved by decreasing the frequency of breathes during IMV or SIMV reducing the pressure during the assist control mode.
3. The patient sits in a chair with arm rests or sits upright in bed.
4. Humidified oxygen or CPAP is prepared if oxygen is connected by a T-piece, extension tubing of 30 cm long should be attached to the exit to prevent entrainment of room air in case the patients inspiratory flow exceed the system flow rate.
5. The air is suctioned.
6. The patient is disconnected from the ventilator, given oxygen or CPAP, encouraged to breathe and monitored for signs of labored breathing, anxiety, desaturation, fatigue or drowsiness.
7. Difficulty in weaning may be due to undetected diaphragmatic paralysis, anxiety or inspiratory muscle fatigue. Reassurance and relaxation feedback can be used for anxiety and periods of rest for fatigue.
8. Preparation with inspiratory muscle training or incentive spirometry is helpful in appropriate patient.

Extubation

After weaning from the ventilator, the endotracheal tube should be removed at the earliest because breathing through an artificial airway can double the load applied to the system. Patients can be extubated once they are alert, able to control their airway, show a stable breathing pattern. The ability to straight leg raise indicates that they have the strength for an effective cough.

Steps for extubation
1. Physiotherapy or airway suction is required.
   a. Check for the cough reflex.
   b. Ensure that reintubation equipment and personnel are available.
   c. Explain the procedure.
   d. Suck out the mouth and throat to clear secretions that they have pooled above the inflated cuff.
   e. Cut the tape holding tube in place, insert a fresh catheter to reach just distal to the tip of the tube deflate cuff, remove tube at peak inspiration when vocal cords are dilated, suction is performed.
   f. Encourage patient to cough out secretions that have accumulated around the distal end of the tube.
2. Given oxygen or CPAP, observe monitors, listen for stridor.
3. Enjoy the patients delight at renewed voice.
4. If sputum retention is anticipated, it better goes for mini-tracheostomy or leads to respiratory distress.

Removal of the Tracheostomy Tube—Postextubation Care

Weaning for tracheostomized patient is to replace the cuffed tube with an uncuffed or fenestrated tube both of which can be played for increasingly longer periods to test for adequate breathing and coughing. The fenestrated tube has an inner and outer cannulae opening in their posterior walls allowing air to pass through the larynx for speech.

Another device is the speaking tube, which is an inner cannula with a flange that closes on expiration thus forcing air through the cords for speech. When the tube has been removed, the patient is taught to hold a sterile dressing firmly over the stoma when coughing.

Myocardial Infarction—Management and Physical Therapy Intervention

CHAPTER 6

MYOCARDIAL INFARCTION

Definition

Myocardium means heart muscle and infarction means death of the tissues. Myocardial infarction means changes occurring in the myocardium secondary to decreased blood flow leading to heart attack. It is a medical emergency condition. Myocardial infarction (MI) is decreased blood flow or stoppage of blood flow to the heart leading to heart muscle damage.

Clinical Features

The clinical features of myocardial infarction are chest pain or tightness or pressure in the chest, pain in the arm, neck back. Shortness of breath, tiredness, nausea, cold sweat, feeling faint, tiredness, vomiting, anxiety, cough, heart burn, indigestion. Myocardial infarction can lead to cardiac arrest, cardiogenic shock, heart failure and heart arrhythmias.

Symptoms

- Chest pain—This is abrupt in onset
- Breathlessness
- Vomiting
- The patient collapses and looks pale, cyanosed, restless, excited, and unconscious
- Levine sign: Patient can localize the chest pain using fists on their sternum

Signs

- Pulse: Fast and feeble
- Blood pressure: Increases
- Heart sounds: Muffled
- Murmurs
- Fever
- Pericardial rub may appear

Risk Factors

The risk factors are obesity, smoking, high total cholesterol includes high triglycerides, high LDL (low density lipids) and low HDL (high density lipids), diabetes, high blood pressure, excess alcohol intake and poor diet.

Pathology: The common pathology is caused by the atherosclerotic plaque formation in coronary artery leads to occlusion and rupture of artery causing coronary thrombosis. Coronary thrombosis causes myocardial tissue damage due to hypoxia and prolonged ischemia.

Diagnosis

Nonspecific Tests

The following are the diagnostic categories. The diagnosis is based on history of the present illness and following tests:
- Cardiac enzymes or cardiac biomarkers. There are 3 cardiac enzymes. They are troponin, myoglobin and creatine kinase. When there is myocardial necrosis the cardiac enzymes are released into the blood circulation and seen in the myocardial infarction. The troponin and creating kinase are elevated.
- Electrocardiogram (ECG): ECG readings are shown as ST segment elevation and T wave inversion.
- Chest X-ray helps to know the size of the heart and blood vessels and also fluid in the lungs.
- Echocardiography helps to detect heart size, shape, and abnormal motion of heart wall.

ECG Changes

ST-segment elevation and T-wave invertion occurs.

Blood Test

Troponin and creatine kinase are elevated.

Echocardiography

Helps to detect heart size, shape, and abnormal motion of heart wall.

Treatment

Medical Treatment

The treatment is divided into conservative and surgical treatment. The conservative treatment is using medication and for complicated myocardial infarction surgical intervention is performed.

Myocardial Infarction—Management and Physical Therapy Intervention

Conservative treatment using medications: The medications prescribed are aspirin for immediate treatment because aspirin helps to reduce blood clots blocking the coronary artery during acute heart attack. Nitroglycerin for the chest pain, anticoagulants like heparin, warfarin (coumadin) to reduce thrombophlebitis and pulmonary embolism, thrombolytic agents are clot busting agents help to dissolve the clot. The medications used are streptase, eminase, etc. and finally aspirin, beta blockers (helps to reduce the blood pressure. The drugs are propranolol and atenolol and statin medication are used to decrease the cholesterol level. They are atorvastatin, provastin. So these medications are prescribed for long term use.

Surgical Treatment

Supplemental oxygen is given for the patient with shortness of breath.

ST-segment elevation myocardial infarction (STEMI): It is a serious heart condition where coronary artery is completely blocked and the heart muscle is not able to receive blood supply so surgical treatment is done. Percutaneous coronary intervention is done where stent is placed to open the arteries and blood supply to the heart muscle is restored.

Non-ST segment myocardial infarction (NSTEMI): This is not a serious condition so heparin medication is prescribed. If the patient is diabetic and has multiple coronary artery blocks then CABG is performed. It is coronary artery bypass surgery.

If there is left ventricular failure then following drugs are prescribed: Diuretics—lower blood pressure, e.g., lasix. Vasodilators relax the smooth muscle in blood vessels causes blood vessels to dilate causing decreased blood pressure, e.g., benazepril. Beta blockers are used to dilate the blood vessels and decrease heart rate and blood pressure. Prescribed for patients with hypertension and arrhythmia.

Common causes that causes loss of life are:
1. First few hours—ventricular fibrillation
2. First few days—pump failure
3. First few months—reinfarction.

Complications
- Atrial fibrillation
- Ventricular tachycardia

- Heart block cause disturbance in heart rhythm
- Stroke
- Cardiogenic shock
- Mitral valve regurgitation
- Pericarditis
- Heart failure.

Surgery

- Percutaneous transluminal coronary angioplasty (PTCA)
- CABG.

Prevention

Primary Prevention

The primary prevention of heart disease are lifestyle modification by the following:
- Smoking cessation and alcohol
- Eat healthy diet and maintain healthy weight
- Regular workout for 5 to 7 days
- Regular physical activity
- Regular follow up.

Secondary Prevention

Regularly follow up with the doctor and using prescribed medications for blood pressure, cholesterol medications like statins lowers cholesterol, aspirin for reducing the blood clot, nitroglycerin for chest pain, etc.

Defibrillator: Defibrillator is an electrical device inserted surgically under the skin for a patient who is medically unstable like signs of heart failure, arrhythmia. This device is connected to the heart and activates with signs of heart failure and derives an electrical shock to prevent arrhythmia.

Cardiac Rehabilitation Exercise Program

The cardiac rehabilitation programme is given to the patient in four phases: They are:
1. Phase-I or Inpatient cardiac rehabilitation
2. Phase-II or Convalescent stage and recovery stage
3. Phase-III or Maintenance stage
4. Phase-IV or Commitment phase.

Myocardial Infarction—Management and Physical Therapy Intervention

Phase-I or Inpatient Cardiac Rehabilitation

The cardiac rehabilitation program is given to the patient when the patient is still in the hospital.

Aims of Phase-I
- To make the patient to return back to early physical activity
- To perform the activities of daily living
- To prevent deep vein thrombosis
- To prevent the effects of the bed rest
- To relieve from anxiety and depression
- To educate both patient and family
- To reduce the risk factors.

Plans of Phase-I
- Regularly monitor the patient's heart rate, blood pressure.
- Initially when the patient is in bed and unable to perform range of motion exercises then passive range of motion exercises are suggested and once the patient is able to perform then active range of motion exercises and finally resisted exercises using weights and Theraband and depending on the patient. All the exercises are performed for bilateral upper extremity and lower extremity to prevent thrombus formation and improve the strength and endurance of the patient.
- Ankle and foot exercises for improving blood supply ,prevent venous pooling and thrombus formation in both lower extremities.
- Breathing exercises to improve breathing pattern, chest mobility and prevent collections of secretions.
- Walking 50 to 75 feet to improve circulation, strengthen muscles and support joints.
- Low level exercise test should be taken to identify patient risk and reduce cardiac mortality rate. During the rest the vital signs are monitored like blood pressure, oxygen saturation levels and heart rate.
- Activities of daily living for day-to-day training and toilet training.
- Progression from 1.0 to 4.0 MET. The exercise starts at 1 MET and depending on the patient tolerance level should be able to progress to 4.0 MET level by end of phase 1.
- Nutritional management with a diet plan is important for healthy weight loss and proper dietary intake.
- Ruling out the risk factors is most important as patient and family has to be educated and patient is also trained for self monitoring of vital signs

- Lifestyle modifications are important to prevent cardiac mortality
- Habits like cessation of the smoking and alcohol consumption
- Recreational interest likes participation in community services for socialization
- Vocational information like type of work, number of hours of work per week, type of job and work related pressure are to be discussed with a professionals and plan accordingly
- Exercise programmer started from the distal to intermediate to the proximal parts of the body and extremities
- Initially exercise both upper extremities and lower extremities followed by trunk
- Exercises are performed in all positions like supine lying, side lying, sitting and standing
- Increased ambulation distance slow and steady to burn more calories and increase functional exercise capacity
- Stair climbing both ascending and descending stair. Start with less number and proceed. Practice according to the patient home environment with or without handrails and no of flights of steps.
- Exercise prescription initially for 5 to 10 minutes for 2 to 4 repetitions and later 20 to 30 minutes for 1 to 2 repetitions.
- Exercise sessions include warm up, endurance aerobic activity and cool down session.

Steps or Levels of Activity for Phase 1

There are 7 steps:

Step-1
- Active and passive range of motion exercises to the extremities
- Ankle and toe exercises done regularly every one hour
- The patient sits in the chair for 15 minutes, 1-2 times per day
- Self care is taught
- Education about intensive care unit, emergencies and services.

Step-2
- Active range of motion exercises to all extremities
- The patient will be sitting on the side of the bed
- The patient sits in the chair for 15-30 minutes for 2-3 times a day
- Complete self care is taught
- Education about role of physiotherapy and cessation of the smoking.

Step-3
- The patient is shifted to the ward
- Ward exercises are taught like warm up exercises
- Exercise done at 2 MET

Myocardial Infarction—Management and Physical Therapy Intervention

- Stretching is taught
- Walking at a slow pace of about 50 feet front and back
- Sitting in a chair
- The patient attends the ward classes in the wheel chair
- The patient walks in the room
- The education is about atherosclerosis, myocardial infarction and 1-2 MET activity.

Step-4
- Range of motion exercises are taught
- Exercise done at 2.5 MET
- The patient walks 75 feet
- The patient is taught the pulse checking and monitoring
- The patient walks to the toilet
- The patient is educated about the risk factors and control.

Step-5
- The range of motion exercises are taught
- The exercise of 3.5 MET is taught
- The patient is taught the pulse checking and monitoring
- The patient walks outside the ward till the corridor
- The patient is educated about the diet, energy conservation during work.

Step-6
- All the above
- Patient ascends and descends the stairs
- The patient walks 500 feet
- Home program is given
- The resident also gets occupational therapy that basically focuses on strengthening of upper extremity. Occupational therapist helps patients to improve, recover, develops and maintains the skills for ADL like dressing, cooking, eating and drinking. OT focuses on residents with sensory, cognitive, physical disabilities be as independent as possible.
- The patient is educated about the drug to be taken and kept with the patient always in emergency of the second attack with emphasis upon exercises, surgery and role of the family for the patient.

Step-7
- All the above
- The patient climb the stairs
- The patient walks about 500 feet
- Home exercises is taught

- Continue with the previous ward activities
- Education about the discharge, medication, diet, exercise regime, back to work, fixing an appointment and review.

Phase -II or Convalescent Stage and Recovery Stage

This is the period from discharge to 12 weeks or 3 months. The patient will be discharged.

Aims of this Phase-II
- To improve the aerobic endurance
- To encourage the patient for positive lifestyle changes
- To promote early return to the normal activity
- To improve the functional capacity
- To educate the patient.

The exercise program is designed based on the graded exercise test and the level of risk factors.

The risk factors affect is as follows:
- *Low risk:* The patient is in uncomplicated zone.
- *Moderate risk or intermediate risk:* The patient has new attack of angina pectoris.
- *High risk:* The patient had attack of recurrent ischemic pain.

In the phase – II, the exercise program depends on intensity of exercise, duration, frequency, mode of exercise according to age, sex and musculoskeletal system. When the patient is given the exercise regime 5 points are checked regularly. They are heart rate, blood pressure, ECG, heart sounds, oxygen saturation and their normal and abnormal values, signs and symptoms. Before prescribing the low to moderate MET the exercise regimen is given and this program should not produce cardiovascular complications or interfere with healing process.

Recovery period: This is the termination of the phase II. The duration is 6-8 weeks. The exercise test is performed. The exercise level is increased.

Phase-III or Maintenance Stage or Maintenance Program

Aim
- To maintain practice and maintain healthy behavior
- To educate on risk factors or risk factors modification
- To become perfect with the exercise program.

Exercise regimen
- The duration of the exercise is for 45 to 60 minutes
- The frequency of the exercise is everyday to the three times a day
- Community exercise program

Myocardial Infarction—Management and Physical Therapy Intervention

- The patient should have the ability to self-regulate exercises
- The functional capacity is about 6 MET.

Phase –IV or Commitment Phase or Ongoing for the Life Phase

The phase is commitment towards the cardiac care like exercises, diet and behavioral modification.

Exercise regimen:
Lifelong commitment to healthy lifestyle, diet management, exercise program and emergency management.

Physical Therapy Treatment at Hospital

After surgery, usually after one day, once the patient is stabilized; simple range of motion exercises are initiated usually in sitting position by lifting legs and arms; vital signs are monitored throughout the session such as blood pressure, heart rate, oxygen levels followed by ambulation program is initiated.

Physical Therapy Program at Outpatient Setting

This is started 4–6 weeks after surgery. Patient needs initial evaluation. Risk factors are monitored such as blood pressure, smoking, body weight, and lipid profile. Exercise stress test is performed to diagnose the patient safety to perform exercise and then exercise program is designed. Goals are established, risk factors are addressed, vital signs are monitored before, during, at the end of the session.

Rehabilitation program includes physical therapy, occupational therapy, and speech therapy. Patient has been evaluated and assessment is done and patient is put on a specific therapy program based on the requirement of the patient and evaluated every 2–4 weeks to know the progress.

Rehabilitation improves cardiac fitness, quality of life, physical exercise capacity, and helps in achieving a healthy and normal lifestyle.

Chronic Obstructive Airway Disease—Management and Physical Therapy Intervention

7

1. Chronic bronchitis
2. Emphysema
3. Asthma
4. Bronchiectasis
5. Cystic fibrosis

■ CHRONIC OBSTRUCTIVE PULMONARY DISEASE

Definition

The chronic obstructive pulmonary disease (COPD) is a chronic, slow progressive disorder characterized by airflow obstruction.

Chronic obstructive pulmonary disease comprises of chronic bronchitis, emphysema, asthma, bronchiectasis, and cystic fibrosis.

Etiology

- Cigarette smoking causes airway inflammation causing a direct imbalance in oxidant/antioxidant capacity and proteinase/antiproteinase level in the lungs.
- Dusty or polluted environment.
- Low birth weight.
- One of the reason for causing emphysema a lung disorder is deficiency of alpha antitrypsin that is genetic protein.

Pathology

- Retention of secretion
- Bronchospasm
- Pulmonary embolus
- Cardiac failure
- Rib fracture—intercostal tears
- Pneumothorax
- CNS depression

Treatment

- Reduction of bronchial irritation

- The respiratory tract infections are treated using antibiotics
- Bronchodilators
- Oxygen therapy
- Anti-inflammatory therapy

Surgical Treatment

Lung transplantation

Complications

- Respiratory failure
- Pneumothorax
- Cor pulmonale
- Heart failure

Prognosis

The prognosis is age related. Patients have better survival rate than those who are suffering from pulmonary hypertension as seen in chronic obstructive pulmonary disease.

CHRONIC BRONCHITIS

Definition

It is a chronic or recurrent increase of mucus secretion on most days for a period of at least three consecutive months of two successive years sufficient to cause expectoration is called chronic expectoration.

Etiology

Age: Middle to adult life
Sex: Men:women = 5:1
Causes: Atmospheric pollution by coal dust or by cigarette smoking.

Pathology

Excess of mucous is produced by irritative substances which stimulates over activity of the mucous secreting glands and goblet cells in the bronchi and bronchioles. The cells increase in size, ducts become dilated and causes chronic inflammatory process which results in mucosal edema that leads to decrease in diameter of airways. Airway obstruction occurs during expiration which results in air-trapping in the alveoli. Lung elasticity is decreased as disease progresses.

Clinical Features

- Initially the cough is intermittent and as condition progresses the cough becomes continuous. In later stages cough is seen in the morning and during lying down
- Sputum will be mucoid and tenacious
- Wheeze will be worse in the morning
- Dyspnea
- Deformity such as barrel chest
- Cyanosis
- Cor pulmonale.

Diagnosis

- X-ray: No abnormality is seen.
- Lung function test: Residual volume and vital capacity is increased, decrease of forced expiratory volume in 1 second (FEV1) and forced vital capacity (FVC) ratio.
- Blood gases: Partial pressure of carbon dioxide increases and partial pressure of oxygen falls.
- Auscultation: Breath sounds are vesicular with prolonged expiration.

Treatment

- Advising the patient to stop smoking, avoiding dusty atmosphere, and if required changing of occupation and housing condition can decrease bronchial irritation.
- The infection should be controlled by antibiotics prescription and during winter the flu season the flu shot should be taken as a preventive measure.
- Control bronchospasm with drugs such as salbutamol.
- Control or decrease the amount of sputum by inhalations and humidification.
- Oxygen therapy: Controlled oxygen is given through ventilatory mask.

Screening and Prevention

a. Avoid smoking as it is one of the leading causes for chronic obstructive lung disease pulmonary.
b. When the patients with chronic bronchitis smoke, it leads to severe illness, shortens lifespan and causes death
c. The patient with chronic bronchitis should stay away from airway pollution, dust at home and workplace or will aggravate the symptoms.

Physical Therapy Intervention

The physical therapy Intervention plays important role for chronic bronchitis patient as it helps keeping air passages free of mucus.
The following techniques are taught to the patient, family or caregiver:
- **Postural drainage:** This is the technique which allows the draining of the secretions from different lobes of the lung and makes secretions to cough out easily.
- **Chest percussion:** This technique includes clapping and percussion on back and chest helps to dislodge the secretions.
- **Coughing techniques:** This helps to cough the secretion out.
- **Breathing exercises:** These are the exercises, which help for breathing with less effort, helps to get more oxygen to the lungs and also strengthening breathing muscles like diaphragm and accessory muscles.
- **Chest wall mobility exercises:** These exercises are important because they help to improve the lungs ventilation.
- **Aerobic exercises:** The aerobic exercises helps in over all functional mobility of the body. They are walking, bicycling (both stationary or outdoor), etc.

EMPHYSEMA

Definition

This is a lung condition with permanent dilatation of the airspaces and destruction of the wall of airways distal to the terminal bronchioles.

Etiology

1. Family history
2. Smoking
3. Congenital factors: Antitrypsin deficiency
4. Secondary to other COPD conditions
5. Pneumoconiosis
6. Sex: Both
7. Age: 40–60 years

Types

1. Centrilobular (centriacinar): Affects only respiratory bronchioles
2. Panacinar (panlobular): Alveoli and respiratory bronchioles.

Clinical Features

1. Dyspnea: Initially on exertion, later on less activity and rest
2. Respiratory pattern: Inspiration is fish like, expiration is pursed lips

3. Cough with sputum
4. Poor posture: Thoracic kyphosis causes elevated and protracted shoulder girdle
5. Cor pulmonale
6. Polycythemia

Diagnosis

1. Breathe sound decreases
2. Prolonged expiration is seen
3. Radiograph: Low and flat diaphragm
4. Chest shape: Barrel chest
5. Lung function tests: FEV1/FEV below 70%, residual volume is increased

Complications

1. Pneumothorax
2. Respiratory failure
3. Congestive cardiac failure

Treatment

1. Every winter as a precautionary measure the flu shot should be taken
2. Antibiotics
3. Stop smoking
4. Change of house, occupation
5. Improve lung function: Steroids, bronchodilators, oxygen therapy.

Surgery

Large bullae are resected to improve lung function.

Prognosis

Emphysema makes patient disabled and causing respiratory failure leading to death.

Physical Therapy Management

The physical therapy management for emphasis focuses basically on three aspects. They are reducing breathlessness, improving strength and endurance and energy conservation. The patient will avoid physical activity because they are physically limited. But encourage patient to participate in physical activities that can improve physical well being and health.

- **Breathing exercises:** The patient is taught breathing exercises and correct breathing pattern to prevent breathlessness.
- **Chest mobility:** The chest mobility exercises are important to maintain correct pattern of breathing.
- **Strength and endurance:** Exercise regime for upper body and lower body strengthening exercises will help to stay fit and health.
- **Energy conservation:** The patient is taught energy conservation to decrease the fatigue levels and improve the performance.

ASTHMA

Definition

Wheezing and breathlessness due to narrowing of the intrapulmonary airways characterize this condition.

Etiology

Common in children. In males, it occurs in childhood, puberty, and later life; in women, it occurs in the middle age.

Types

Extrinsic and intrinsic asthma.

Extrinsic or Atopic Asthma

This occurs in the younger groups.

Etiology: Allergic pollen, house mites, feathers, food, fur, drugs, and family history.

Pathology: Exposure causes mucosal inflammatory allergic changes and asthma will be episodic.

Onset: Sudden, paroxysmal, night.

Symptoms
- Chest tightness, dryness or irritation in the upper respiratory track
- Attack: Episodic
- Duration: Few seconds to months
- Severity: Mild wheezing to great distress

Clinical features
1. Wheeze and dyspnea
2. Cough
3. Posture

4. Pulse: Rapid, paradoxical
5. Tachycardia
6. Cyanosis
7. Breath sounds: Vesicular with prolonged expiration and high-pitched rhonchi
8. Percussion: Hyper-resonant

Diagnosis
- Radiograph: Chest will be overshaded.
- Lung function test: FEV1 and FEV drop on severe attack.

Intrinsic Asthma or Nonatopic Asthma

Age: The intrinsic asthma or nonatopic asthma is a chronic condition that is commonly seen in older adults.

Etiology
1. Bronchial infection
2. Chronic bronchitis
3. Strenuous exercise
4. Stress or anxiety

Pathology: Main pathological changes occurring during an asthmatic attack are as follows:
1. Spasm of the smooth muscle in the walls of the bronchi and bronchioles
2. Edema of the mucous membrane of the bronchi and bronchioles
3. Excessive mucus production

Clinical features
1. Associated with chronic bronchitis
2. Wheeze and dyspnea are continuous and worse in the morning
3. Cough produces mucoid sputum
4. Respiratory infection occurs

Diagnosis
Radiograph: This shows emphysematous changes.

Status Asthmaticus: This is the severe progressive acute attack of asthma usually present for 24 hours and is a life-threating condition. Status asthmaticus also called severe asthma exacerbation or acute severe asthma. The symptoms include shortness of breath, anxiety and fatigue this condition does not respond to the bronchodilators. It leads to respiratory failure and patient has to seek medical treatment.

Treatment

Aim
1. Prevention of attack
2. Maintenance of general fitness
3. Treatment during an attack

Management
1. Patient should be careful with the diet so few foods may aggravate the asthma symptoms, home environment should be dust free, avoid pets because pet hair can induce asthma symptoms, adequate ventilation also helps as fresh air prevents infections like bronchitis, asthma. The patient should also be free of stress and anxiety.
2. Drugs: Administration of medicine using aerosol is effective for longer duration like using bronchodilators for wheezing, corticosteroids should be used if bronchodilators are not effective. Rotahalers and Spinhalers deliver the drug in dry powdered form.

Physical Therapy Management

The patient is focused on the following breathing exercises, inspiratory muscle training:

- Airway clearance techniques, physical techniques. All these help the patient to improve the quality of the life, reduced anxiety and depression, lower medication use and improve cardiopulmonary fitness.
- **Breathing exercises:** The patient is taught diaphragmatic breathing and nasal breathing. Patient should be practicing slow breathing pattern rate with longer duration of expiration so reducing residual volume.
- **Inspiratory muscle training:** The patient is taught this technique using an external resistive device. This technique improves strength and endurance of the inspiratory muscles and chest muscles so can improve the exercise tolerance and decrease the episodes of dyspnea.
- **Physical fitness:** The asthma patient does not participate in physical fitness and sports programs secondary to fear of breathlessness so patients are specially designed with physical fitness program to overcome the fear and decrease breathlessness.
- **Airway clearance techniques:** The patient and the family are trained with airway clearance techniques for sputum mobilization. Some of them are postural drainage using percussion and clapping techniques and coughing techniques.

BRONCHIECTASIS

Definition

It is an abnormal dilatation of the bronchi associated with obstruction and infection.

Etiology

Congenital

This is rare and occurs in triad. They are frontal sinusitis, visceral transposition, and bronchiectasis.

Acquired

The causes are bronchial obstruction, bacterial infection, tumor or foreign body.

Clinical Features

1. Whooping cough
2. Measles
3. Pneumonia

Site: This is bilateral and affects lower lobes.

Pathology

Bronchial obstruction will cause absorption of the air from the lung tissue making the airway shrink and collapse, hence there is increase in load of proximal airways which can get distort and dilated. Secretions gets accumulated and infected, pus is formed. The mucosal lining is replaced by granulation tissue so mucous passage is hindered. Hemoptysis occurs as a result of arterial vessels anastomosis with the pulmonary capillaries.

Clinical Features

Onset: Childhood
1. Cough—Persistent
2. Sputum: Purulent sputum, green in color, foul smell
3. Dyspnea
4. Hemoptysis
5. Recurrent pneumonia
6. Halitosis
7. Chronic sinusitis

8. Pyrexia
9. Night sweats
10. Anorexia
11. Malaise
12. Weight loss
13. Lassitude
14. Clubbing
15. Decrease in thoracic mobility.

Investigations

- **Radiograph:** Bronchovascular markings are seen, multiple cysts with fluid levels are seen.
- **Bronchography:** This is the diagnostic test for radiographic imaging using opaque substance. The test provides details of the respiratory tree. Recently this test is rarely performed and improved by using bronchoscopy and computed tomography.
- **Sputum culture:** *Haemophilus influenzae, Staphylococcus.*

Complications

1. Recurrent hemoptysis
2. Pleurisy and empyema
3. Abscess formation
4. Emphysema
5. Respiratory failure
6. Right ventricular failure
7. Pneumonia

Treatment

1. Relieve obstruction
2. Control infection by antibiotics
3. Good diet and fresh air for promoting good health

Surgery

1. Segmental resection
2. Lobectomy

Physical Therapy Management

The physical therapy management focuses on increasing aerobic capacity, active cycle of breathing techniques, positive expiratory pressure, autogenic drainage, oscillative expiratory positive pressure, high frequency chest wall oscillation.

The patient is taught about importance of aerobic exercise like walking, biking, etc. as it improves endurances, reduces the episode of dyspnea and fatigue. Active cycle of breathing techniques is three phases of breathing exercises, which helps to clear the secretions from lungs. In the first phase relax your airways, in the second phase the mucus clearance occurs and in the third phase mucus is forced out of the lungs.

- **Positive expiratory pressure:** In this the patient expires through a mask against the resistance. This techniques improves ventilation, clears secretions from lungs, prevent air trapping.
- **Autogenic drainage or self drainage:** It is independent airway clearance technique, which teaches patient using different speeds of breathing to bring the secretions outside.
- **Oscillating expiratory positive pressure:** It is a technique used with aero eclipse breath actuated nebulizer, which helps to loosen and removal of the lung secretions.

High frequency chest wall oscillation is a airway clearance technique where outside or external chest wall oscillations applied using a vest around the chest wall where different parameters are applied to loosen and expel the mucus out of the lungs.

CYSTIC FIBROSIS OR MUCOVISCIDOSIS

Definition

Cystic fibrosis is the condition where there is disorder of exocrine glands with a high sodium chloride content in the sweat and pancreatic insufficiency causing malabsorption syndrome.

Etiology

Heredity.

Pathology

Pulmonary changes:
a. The pulmonary changes seen in cystic fibrosis are excessive mucus production in bronchi and bronchioles and blocked by mucus plugs.
b. **Viscid mucus:** The mucous produced will be viscid and sticks to the bronchial walls.

c. **Infection:** When the mucus gets infected by the bacteria, the secretion's become purulent leading to inflammation and irritation of the bronchial wall tissues.
d. **Bronchiectasis:** Bronchiectasis is a lung condition where the weakening and dilatation of the bronchial walls occurs.
e. **Abnormal development of the lung tissue:** The excessive mucus production and blocking by mucus plugs, infection by the bacteria causing inflammation of the bronchial wall, bronchiectasis all leads to abnormal development of the lung tissue.

Clinical Features

S. No.	Children	S. No.	Adolescents and adults
1.	Meconium ileus	1.	Breathlessness
2.	Foul smelling stools	2.	Wheezing
3.	Sweating	3.	Productive cough
4.	Wheeze	4.	Purulent sputum
5.	Dyspnea	5.	Hemoptysis
6.	Under weight	6.	Finger clubbing
7.	Cough	7.	Puberty changes
		8.	Infertility in males
		9.	Respiratory failure
		10.	Cyanosis
		11.	Cor pulmonale

Complications

- Hemoptysis
- Spontaneous pneumothorax
- Lung abscess
- Bronchiectasis
- Liver disease
- Psychosocial disturbance

Treatment

1. Antibiotics
2. Bronchodilators
3. Oxygen therapy
4. A low-fat high-calorie diet is recommended supplemented with vitamins
5. Pancreatic enzymes are given before each meal to improve absorption

Physical Therapy Treatment for Cystic Fibrosis

S. No.	Aims of physical therapy	Plans of physical therapy
1.	To improve breathing efficiency	Deep breathing exercises
2.	To increase activity tolerance, functional capacity and energy conservation	Activity pacing, balance rest and activities
3.	To drain the secretions	Postural drainage, percussion, vibration and clapping
4.	To remove the secretions	Coughing, huffing techniques
5.	To teach home exercise program	Active cycle of breathing techniques

Cardiac Rehabilitation 8

INTRODUCTION

Cardiac rehabilitation is a multidisciplinary program for patients with heart disease to achieve physical, psychological, and functional status and to improve the quality of life.

The cardiac rehabilitation is a long-term comprehensive rehabilitation program with graded exercise. This results in improvement of physical, physiological, and psychological well-being of the patient. It is a successful measure in lowering mortality rate in patients suffering from cardiac disease.

AIMS OF CARDIAC REHABILITATION

1. To help the individual regain strength
2. To improve functional capacity
3. To encourage exercise training
4. To prevent the reversal of the symptoms
5. To maximize the cardiac function
6. To build fitness and functional capacity
7. To prevent worsening of the symptoms
8. To reduce the risk of future heart problems
9. To improve health and maintain the quality of life
10. To mold the patient's lifestyle and habits such as smoking cessation
11. To bring changes in the diet by attending the nutritional classes
12. To teach stress management techniques and techniques to reduce the anxiety
13. To counsel and educate the patient about the heart condition and its management
14. To encourage and prepare the patient to return to the work and meet the demands of the job both physically and psychologically

TEAM OF THE CARDIAC REHABILITATION PROGRAM

The cardiac rehabilitation program is conducted for both inpatients and outpatients. The skilled professional team includes:
1. Cardiologist
2. Cardiovascular surgeon

3. Dietician
4. Physical therapist
5. Occupational therapist
6. Speech therapist
7. Psychiatrist
8. Rehabilitation nurse

INDICATIONS OF THE CARDIAC REHABILITATION PROGRAM

1. Myocardial infarction
2. Angina pectoris
3. Coronary artery bypass surgery
4. Valve transplant
5. Heart failure
6. Heart transplant
7. Angioplasty
8. High-risk patient
9. Congestive heart failure
10. Congenital heart disease
11. Open-heart surgery
12. Angina
13. Arrhythmias
14. Balloon angioplasty
15. Rheumatic heart disease.

CONTRAINDICATIONS

1. Hypertension
2. Diabetes mellitus
3. Congestive heart failure
4. Acute illness
5. Angina.

CATEGORIES OF CARDIAC REHABILITATION PROGRAM

Cardiac rehabilitation is divided into two categories:
1. Inpatient
2. Outpatient: This category is in turn divided into three phases:
    a. Convalescent/recovery phase
    b. Maintenance phase
    c. Commitment phase

CARDIAC REHABILITATION EXERCISE PROGRAM

The cardiac rehabilitation program is divided into four phases:
1. Phase-I or inpatient cardiac rehabilitation
2. Phase-II or convalescent stage and recovery stage
3. Phase-III or maintenance stage
4. Phase-IV or commitment phase.

Phase-I or Inpatient Cardiac Rehabilitation

The cardiac rehabilitation program is given to the patient when the patient is still in the hospital.

Aims of Phase-I

1. To make the patient to return to early physical activities.
2. To perform the activities of dailylife
3. To prevent deep vein thrombosis
4. To prevent the effects of bed rest
5. To relieve from anxiety and depression
6. To educate both patient and family
7. To reduce the risk factors

Plans of Phase-I

1. Regularly monitor the patient's heart rate, blood pressure
2. Initially passive range-of-motion exercises, then active exercises, and finally resisted exercises
3. Ankle and foot exercises
4. Breathing exercises
5. Walking 50–75 ft.
6. Low-level exercise test
7. Activities of daily living training and toilet training
8. Progression from 1.0 to 4.0 maximal exercise test (MET)
9. Nutritional management with a diet plan
10. Ruling out the risk factors
11. Lifestyle modifications
12. Habits such as cessation of the smoking
13. Recreational interest
14. Vocational information such as type of work, number of hours of work per week, type of job, and work-related pressure
15. Exercise program: The exercises should begin with the extremities. In the upper extremity start with finger, wrist, forearm, elbow, shoulder and shoulder girdle and in lower limb start with toes, foot ankle, knee, hip

16. Initially exercises performed in the extremities followed by exercises to trunk are performed
17. Exercises in supine lying, side lying, sitting, and standing
18. Increased ambulation
19. Stair climbing both ascending and descending
20. Exercise prescription initially for 5-10 minutes for 2-4 repetitions and later 20-30 minutes for 1-2 repetitions
21. Exercise sessions include warm-up, endurance aerobic activity, and cooldown session

Steps or Levels of Activity for Phase-I

There are seven steps:

Step-1
In the step one the focus is on range of motion exercises. Depending on the muscle grade the range of motion exercise are performed.
1. Manual muscle testing grades and range of motion exercises prescribed:
   Grade zero: None: No visible contraction or palpation available so passive rage of motion is performed to all extremities.
   Grade one: Trace: Palpable or visible contraction is seen but no motion can be performed by the patient so passive range of motion is performed to all extremities.
   Grade two: Poor: Full range of motion exercises can be performed in the gravity eliminate so active assisted exercises are performed to all the extremities.
   Grade Three: Fair: Full range of motion exercises can be performed against the gravity so resistive exercises can be performed with minimal resistant like using Theraband exercises to all extremities.
   Grade Four: Good: Full range of motion exercises can be performed against the gravity using moderate resistance like using weights raging from 1 pound to 2.5 pounds depending on patients.
   Grade Five: Normal: Full range of motion exercises can be performed against the gravity using maximum resistance like using weights ranging from 3 pound to 5 pounds depending on patients tolerance and also precautions, indications and contraindications are to be considered before giving weights to the patient tolerance and also precautions, indications and contraindications are to be considered before giving weights to the patient.

2. Ankle and toe exercises done regularly if possible more often. These exercises help to strengthen and stretch the foot muscles, these exercises are highly recommended for peripheral neuropathy pain relief, prevent toe cramps, prevent heel and arch pain and hammer toes.
3. The patient sits on the chair for 15 minutes, 1-2 times per day. The patient is recommended to avoid laying in the bed for longer duration and recommended to sit on the chair as often as possible to prevent bed rest complications.
4. The patient is taught performing self-care like feeding, combing hair, upper and lower body dressing, toileting and transfers and wheel chair mobility if required called activities of daily living. This job is basically done by the occupational therapist
5. Patient and family are education about intensive care unit, emergencies, and services available. The details of the services available and way to approach in case of emergency the details are explained and given by the social workers

Step-2
1. The patient is taught active range of motion exercises to all muscles and joints for 3 sets of 10 repetitions with rest breaks in between the sets and exercises performed to all extremities.
2. The patient is encouraged to sit at the edge of the bed. Check for signs of dizziness, which can be cause of orthostatic hypotension. So patient is taught bed mobility activities like rolling to both the sides in the bed to take away pressure off the back, coming from supine lying to sitting. If patient feels dizzy then patient is encouraged to go to side-lying position and then come to sitting at the edge of the bed.
3. The patient is encouraged to sit more often as lying in the bed may lead to bed rest complications. So patient is encouraged to sit in the chair for 15 to 30 minutes for 2 to 3 times a day.
4. The occupational therapist teaches complete self care like hygiene and grooming, working on strengthening of both the upper extremities and encouraging patient to participate in recreational activities if possible.
5. Patient is educated about cessation of smoking and its effects and complications. Also educate the patient about the importance of physical therapy sessions.

Step-3
1. The patient is shifted to the ward
2. Ward exercises are taught such as warm-up exercises

3. Exercise done at 2 MET
4. Stretching is taught
5. Walking at a slow pace of about 50 ft. front and back
6. Sitting in a chair
7. The patient attends the ward classes in the wheel chair
8. The patient walks in the room
9. The education is about atherosclerosis, myocardial infarction, and 1–2 MET activity

Step-4
1. Range-of-motion exercises are taught
2. Exercise done at 2.5 MET
3. The patient walks 75 ft
4. The patient is taught the pulse checking and monitoring
5. The patient walks to the toilet
6. The patient is educated about the risk factors and control

Step-5
1. The range-of-motion exercises are taught
2. The exercise of 3.5 MET is taught
3. The patient is taught the pulse checking and monitoring
4. The patient walks outside the ward till the corridor
5. The patient is educated about the diet, energy conservation during work

Step-6
1. All the above
2. Patient ascends and descends the stairs
3. The patient walks 500 ft
4. Home program is given
5. The resident also gets occupational therapy (OT) that basically focuses on strengthening of upper extremity. Occupational therapist helps patients to improve, recover, develop, and maintain the skills for activities of daily living (ADL) such as dressing, cooking, eating, and drinking. Occupational therapy focuses on residents with sensory, cognitive, and physical disabilities be as independent as possible.
6. The patient is educated about medications to be taken during the emergency situation and patient always carry the medication with them to use during the emergency situations. The family is also educated about the same.

Step-7
1. All the above
2. The patient climbs the stairs

3. The patient walks about 500 ft
4. Home exercises are taught
5. Continue with the previous ward activities
6. Education about the discharge, medication, diet, exercise regime, back to work, fixing an appointment, and review

Phase-II or Convalescent Stage and Recovery Stage

This is the period from discharge to 12 weeks or 3 months. The patient will be discharged.

Aims of Phase-II

1. To improve the aerobic endurance
2. To encourage the patient for positive lifestyle changes
3. To promote early return to the normal activity
4. To improve the functional capacity
5. To educate the patient

The exercise program is designed based on the graded exercise test and the level of risk factors.

Type of Risks

1. **Low-risk:** The patient is not under any complication.
2. **Moderate or intermediate risk:** The patient has angina pectoris.
3. **High-risk:** The patient had attack of recurrent ischemic pain.

In Phase-II, the exercise program has intensity of exercise, duration, frequency, and mode of exercise according to age, sex, and musculoskeletal system.

When the patient is given the exercise regime, five points are checked regularly: heart rate, blood pressure, ECG, heart sounds, and their signs and symptoms.

Before prescribing the low-to-moderate MET, the exercise regimen is given and this program should not produce cardiovascular complications or interfere with healing process.

Recovery Period

This is the termination of Phase-II. The duration is 6–8 weeks. The exercise test is performed. The exercise level is increased.

Phase-III or Maintenance Stage or Maintenance Program

Aims of Phase-III

1. To maintain the function
2. To educate on risk factors or risk factors modification
3. To become perfect with the exercise program

Exercise Regimen

1. The duration of the exercise is for 45–60 minutes.
2. The frequency of exercise program is 1 to 3 times a day depending on the requirement and patient's medical condition. The total duration of exercise is 45 min to 60 min. So if the patient is doing exercise 3 times a day then the duration can be split into 3 sessions. So patient does not exceed the safe limit of exercise program.
3. Community exercise program.
4. The patient should have the ability to self-regulate exercises.
5. The functional capacity is about 6 MET.

Phase-IV or Commitment Phase or Ongoing for the Life Phase

The phase is commitment toward the cardiac care such as exercises, diet, and behavioral modification.

THE CARDIAC RESPONSE TO THE EXERCISE

1. **Normal response:** Cardiac output, heart rate increases with increase of workload and oxygen consumption. The maximum heart rate decreases, and in the blood pressure, there is rise in systolic blood pressure, whereas the diastolic pressure will rise only slightly.
2. **Abnormal response:** The abnormal response of the Heart is diagnosed based on the following:
   a. *ECG (Electrocardiograph—A diagnostic test):* The elevation or depression of ST segment indicates heart injury. The response seen is either elevation or depression of ST segment in ECG, a diagnostic test indicates heart injury.
   b. *The blood pressure:* The blood pressure is measured as systolic blood pressure by diastolic blood pressure. The normal value is 120/80 mm of Hg. The blood pressure is increased with the exercise. The systolic blood pressure increases but diastolic blood pressure remains the same. But if diastolic blood pressure increases by 15 mm Hg then the valve is considered abnormal and a medical emergency.
   c. *Heart rate:* Heart rate is classified as—bradycardia (decreased heart rate) and tachycardia (elevated heart rate). In bradycardia the resting heart rate is 60 beats per min. This condition only shows symptoms if heart rate is below 50 beats per

Cardiac Rehabilitation

minute. The symptoms will be dizziness, fainting, fatigue, weakness and sweating. In tachycardia the increased heart rate is greater than 100 beats per minute. It is of three types:
  i. Supraventricular tachycardia: The heart beats so fast that ventricles contract before filling. So systemic circulation is decreased.
  ii. Ventricular tachycardia: It is similar to supraventricular tachycardia. The electrical conduction occurs in the wrong direction. So systemic circulation is decreased.
  iii. Sinus tachycardia: Heart is the natural pacemaker but beats faster than the normal rhythm.
3. The blood pressure; the systolic pressure is in the normal level or becomes high after exercise whereas the diastolic pressure increases to 20 mm Hg or it decreases.
4. Angina symptoms: The angina symptoms are following. The patient complains of pain, heaviness and tightness in the chest area, dizziness and fatigue are the common symptoms. This is an emergency situation.

Bradycardia or tachycardia—abnormal exercise

The resident will be assessed first followed by cardiorespiratory fitness test and resident is put on cardiac rehabilitation program based on the results.

Assessment

According to the cardiac disability classification:
- **Class-1:** No symptoms with ordinary physical activity.
- **Class-2:** Symptoms with ordinary activity. There will be slight limitation of the activity.
- **Class-3:** Symptoms with less than ordinary activity and limitation of activity is seen.
- **Class-4:** Symptoms with any physical activity or even at rest.

CARDIORESPIRATORY FITNESS TEST

The fitness evaluation is done on the patient both on rest and during exercise. This measures maximum oxygen uptake denoted by VO_2.

Guidelines

1. Age and risk factors should be considered.
2. One day before the test is done, the therapist must give pretest instructions.

3. The patient is instructed to read and sign the consent form and physical activity readiness questionnaire (PAR-Q).

Procedure

1. Check the patient's resting heart rate and blood pressure.
2. When the test is started, monitor the heart rate and blood pressure and ratings of perceived exertion (RPE) at frequent intervals.
3. Exercise heart rate measured at the end of 1 minute.
4. Blood pressure and RPE are monitored at the end of the stage of exercise.
5. Monitor the patient's physical appearance and symptoms throughout the test.
6. Cooldown exercise is must because active recovery reduces the risk of hypotension.
7. Measure postexercise heart rate, blood pressure, and RPE for ≥4 minutes, if any abnormal responses are seen, measure for longer period.
8. The heart rate and blood pressure during this period should be stable but higher than pre-exercise level.
9. When the patient complaints of discomfort, the patient is asked to sit down. Check the vital signs of the patient and closely monitor the patient for the symptoms.
10. Heart rate is measured pretest, exercise, and recovery periods.

There are two different exertion grade scales. Any one of the scale can be followed. They are described in the following sections.

Ratings of Perceived Exertion Scale

No.	Category scale	No.	Category ratio scale
6	No exertion at all	0	No exertion
7	Extremely light exertion	0.5	Extremely weak exertion
9	Very light exertion	1	Very weak exertion
11	Light exertion	2	Light exertion
13	Somewhat hard exertion	3	Moderate exertion
15	Hard exertion	5	Strong exertion
17	Very hard exertion	7	Very strong exertion
19	Extremely hard exertion	10	Extremely strong exertion
20	Maximal exertion		

Borg 10—Exertion Grade Scale

Grade	Type of exertion
0	No exertion
0.5	Very very weak exertion
1.0	Very weak exertion
1.5	Very light exertion
3.0	Moderate exertion
4.0	Somewhat strong exertion
5.0	Heavy exertion
7.0	Very heavy exertion
10.0	Maximum exertion

Indications for Termination of the Test

1. Onset of angina
2. Decreased blood pressure
3. Excess increase of blood pressure
4. Fatigue
5. Nausea
6. Light-headedness
7. Confusion

Test Termination

The patient voluntarily terminates or the therapist is aware of the indications of the patient from stopping the test by signs and symptoms.

EXERCISE TEST PROTOCOL

1. **Maximal exercise test (MET)**
    a. Treadmill maximal exercise test
    b. Bicycle ergometer maximal exercise test
    c. Bench stepping maximal exercise test
2. **Submaximal exercise test**
    a. Treadmill submaximal exercise test
    b. Bicycle ergometer submaximal exercise test
    c. Bench stepping submaximal exercise test

Maximal Exercise Test

The MET is used to assess the aerobic capacity. Selection of appropriate exercise mode and test protocol required for the patient according to the age, gender, health, and fitness status is done.

Guidelines of Exercise Testing

1. The treadmill or stationary bicycle ergometer for graded exercise testing (GXT).
2. Begin with 2-3-minutes warm-up.
3. The intensity of the exercise should be slow.
4. There should be gradual increase of exercise intensity.
5. For healthy individual, the MET value can be 2 MET and for the disease individual, it can be 0.5 MET.
6. Monitor heart rate each minute of GXT, heart rate should stabilize between two heart rates within ±5-6 beats per minute (bpm).
7. Measure blood pressure and ratings of perceive exertion at each stage of GXT.
8. Check signs and symptoms of the patient, if severe ask patient to terminate the test.
9. For submaximal GXT, heart rate range 70-85% is sufficient and test can be terminated.
10. Cooldown period for about 4 minutes or more is called recovery period. During this period, check heart rate and blood pressure. Passive recovery is used if patient experiences signs of discomfort.
11. Estimate exercise tolerance in MET for treadmill protocol.
12. Testing should be quiet, room temperature of 21-23°C and humidity is 60% or less than that can be considered.

Exercise regime
1. Treadmill walking
2. Running
3. Stationary cycle
4. For paraplegics and patients with limited use of upper extremity, this arm ergometry can be tested
5. For large group, bench stepping can be tested

Maximum exercise testing
1. **Continuous VO_2 maximum test:** This is the test without rest between work.
2. **Discontinuous tests:** This test gives 5-10-minute rest intervals between workload.

Once the test is completed ACSM metabolic equation is used for the clinical testing. This is used to estimate the rate of energy expenditure for treadmill walking, running, bicycle ergometer, and bench stepping test both maximal and submaximal exercise testing. The total energy expenditure is in mL/kg/min.

Cardiac Rehabilitation

There are three functional components: horizontal, vertical, and resting for energy expenditure.

Maximal Exercise Testing

Maximum exercise testing on treadmill: This exercise testing is done on the motorized treadmill. The parameters required are speed of about 25 miles per hour (mph) and inclination–elevation per 100 horizontal units.

Metabolic Calculation

S. No.	VO_2 mode (units)	Resting component→	Horizontal component, H	Vertical component, V
1.	Walking mL/kg/min	3.5 mL/kg/min	Speed (m/min) × 0.1	Grade (decimal) × m/min × 1.8
2.	Running mL/kg/min	3.5 mL/kg/min	Speed (m/min) × 0.2	Grade (decimal) × m/kg/min/min × 0.9
3.	Leg ergometer mL/min	3.5 mL/kg/min × kg BW	None	Kilogram meter per minute × 2
4.	Arm ergometer mL/min	3.5 mL/kg/min × kg BW	None	Kilogram meter per minute × 3
5.	Stepping	Included in H and V components	Steps/min × 0.35	1.33 to 1.81 m/step The positive value is 1.0 m/step The Negative value is 0.33 m/step

Valid Estimation: ACSM Metabolic Equation to Estimate VO_2

1. Body weight (BW) in kg if pound 1 kg = 2.2 lb.
2. Treadmill speed 1 mph = 26.8 m/min.
3. Treadmill grade from percent to decimal.
4. Convert MET to mL/kg/min. 1 MET = 3.5 mL/kg/min.
5. Convert Watts to kgm/min. 1 W = 6 kgm/min.
6. For arm and leg ergometer, it is nonweight-bearing so has to convert mL/kg/min to mL/min.
7. For walking, running and bench stepping, it is weight-bearing so convert mL/min to mL/kg/min.
8. Convert the step height in inches to meter. 1 in.=0.0254 m.

Examples

1. If the BW of the person is 180 lb, then BW in kg is BW in pound/2.2 lb so we can get the BW in kg as 1 kg = 2.2 lb, 180/2.2 = 82 kg.

2. Treadmill speed is 1 mph = 26.8 m/min. The patient speed is calculated with the treadmill speed. If the Patient speed is 6 mph then total speed is 26.8 × 6 mph = 160.8 mph.
3. Treadmill grade from percent to decimal is if percent is 14%, then decimal is 14 × 100 = 0.14.
4. Convert MET to mL/kg/min. 1 MET = 3.5 mL/kg/min. If the patient MET is 6, then 6 × 3.5 = 21 mL/kg/min.
5. Convert Watts to kg-m/min. 1 W = 6 kg-m/min. When there are 140 watts then the conversion of total watts is equal to 8,406 kg-m/min.
6. For arm and leg ergometer, it is nonweight-bearing so has to convert mL/kg/min to mL/min. 30 mL/kg/min × 70 kg = 2,100 mL/min.
7. For walking, running, and bench stepping, it is weight-bearing so convert mL/min to mL/kg/min. 2,400 mL/min/60 kg = 40 mL/kg/min.
8. Convert the step height in inches to meter. 1 in.=0.0254 m. If the step height is 8 in., then 8 in. × 0.0254 = 0.2032 m.

ACSM Walking Equation

VO_2 = Resting component + horizontal component + vertical component

3.5 + speed (m/min) × 0.1 + grade × (decimal) × speed (m/min) × 1.8.

1. Convert the speed in mph to m/min
   1 mph = 26.8 m/min
   2.5 mph × 26.8 = 67 m/min
2. Calculate the horizontal component
   H = speed × 0.1 = 67 m/min × 0.1 = 67 mL/kg/min
3. Calculate the vertical component (V) by converting % grade into the decimal by dividing by 100
   V = grade (decimal) × speed × 1.8
   0.20 × 67 m/min × 1.8 = 24.12 mL/kg/min
4. Calculate the total VO_2 in mL/kg/min by adding the H, V, R components
   R = 1 MET = 3.5 mL/kg/min
   VO_2 = H + V + R = (67 + 24.12 + 3.5) mL/kg/min
   = 94.62 mL/kg/min
5. Calculate the rate of energy expenditure (E) in MET by converting VO_2 to MET
   E = VO_2/1 MET or 3.5 mL/kg/min
   = 94.62 mL/kg/min/3.5 = 27.0 mL/kg/min

Bicycle Ergometer Maximal Exercise Tests

This is the commonly used instrument. There is friction-type bicycle ergometer where the resistance is applied against the flywheel using a belt and weighted pendulums. This bicycle has handwheel that adjusts the workload either by tightening or loosening the brace belt. The workload can be increased by raising the resistance on the flywheel.

Power = force × distance/time
P = Watts. 1 W = 6 kgm/min
Force = kilograms
Distance = number of revolutions per minute
Power = 2 kg × 6 m × 60 rpm = 720 kgm/min or 120 W.

The distance is calculated by measuring the circumference in meters of the resistance track on the flywheel and multiplying the circumference by the number of flywheel revolutions during on complete revolution (360°) of the pedal.

Some ergometers have speedometer that displays the individual pedaling rate. Few use a metronome to establish clients pedaling cadence.

Test protocols
Pedaling ate: 50 or 60 rpm
Power: 150–300 kgm/min (25–50 W)

The total energy expenditure in mL/min is a function of two components.
1. **Vertical component:** The energy expenditure to overcome the resistance of flywheel per minute.
2. **Resting component:** It is the amount of the oxygen consumed per minute by the client at rest and depends on the BW.
   Resting component: Resting metabolic equivalent (1 MET or 3.5 mL/kg/min)

Ergometer—Uses

S. No.	Advantages	Disadvantages
1.	Safer than treadmill	Difficult to calibrate
2.	Easy to monitor	Leg fatigue occurs
3.	Easy to quantify the work	Lower VO_2 maximum
4.	Easy to obtain the details	

ACSM leg ergometer equation
To calculate the energy expenditure of a 60 kg (132 lb) (as 1 kg = 2.2 lb) women cycling at the work rate of 400 kgm/min.

1. Resting component: (V)
   V = kgm/min × 2 = 400 kgm/min × 2 = 800 mL/min
2. Absolute VO_2 = V = + (1 MET × BW = 3.5 mL/kg/min × 60 kg = 210 mL/min)
   VO_2 = 800 mL/min + 210 mL/min = 1,010 mL/min
   Convert the absolute VO_2 to relative VO_2 by dividing the BW
   Relative VO_2 = absolute VO_2/BW
   Relative VO_2 = 1,010 mL/min/60 kg = 16.8 mL/kg/min
   Relative energy expenditure in MET is calculated by dividing 3.5 mL/kg/min.
   MET = 16.8 mL/kg/min/3.5 mL/kg/min = 58.8 MET

Bench Stepping Maximal Exercise Tests

The individual in this type of the test performs up-phase or positive work and down-phase or negative work.

The intensity of the work is increased by gradual increase of the height of the bench or rate of stepping.

Work can be calculated by the equation:
$W = F \times D$
F = body weight in kilograms
D = bench height ties the number of steps per minute

For example, a 60-kg (132 lb) woman stepping at a rate of 20 steps/min on a 25-cm bench.
W = 60 kg × 0.25 × 20 steps/min
= 300 kgm/min.

The negative work is combined with the step height and the rate of stepping in different BWs as less energy consumed in negative work.

The equation to adjust the step height and stepping rate for differences in the BW to achieve a given work rate:

Step height (cm) = work [(kg cm)/min]/body weight (kg) × stepping rate (cm).

Stepping rate (steps/min: = work [(kg cm)/min]/body weight (kg) × step height (cm).

Graded step test protocol:
   Patient = 50 kg (110 lb); work rate = 200 kgm/min
   Stepping rate is set at 16 steps/min.

Step height: Work rate/patient weight × stepping rate = 200 kgm/min/50 kg × 16 steps/min
= 200 kgm/min/800 = 0.25 m or 25 cm.

Stepping rate = work rate/patient weight × step height = 400 kgm/min/50 kg × 0.25 m = 400 kgm/min/12.5 = 32 steps/min.

ACSM Stepping Equation

To calculate the energy expenditure for the bench stepping using a 14-in. step height at a cadence of 22 steps/min.

Follow these steps:
VO_2 = Horizontal component + vertical component
VO_2 in mL/kg/min = (steps/min × 0.35) + (m/step × steps/min × 1.33 × 1.8).

1. Calculate the horizontal component (H)
   H = Stepping rate × 0.35 = 22 steps/min × 0.35 = 7.7 mL/kg/min.
2. To convert the bench height to the meter (1 in. = 2.54 cm or 0.0254 m)
   Height = 14 in. × 0.0254 = 0.3556.
3. To calculate the vertical component (V) the following equation is used: V = Bench height × Stepping rate × 1.33 × 1.8. So 0.3556 (Bench height) × 22 steps/min (Stepping height) × 1.33 × 1.8 = 18.72 mL/kg/min.
4. Add the horizontal component and vertical component to calculate the relative VO_2:
   VO_2 = 7.7 mL/kg/min + 18.72 mL/kg/min = 26.42 mL/kg/min.
5. Convert the VO_2 to MET by dividing by 3.5 mL/kg/min MET = 26.42 mL/kg/min/3.5 mL/kg/min = 7.54 MET.

Submaximal Exercise Test

This consists of the following tests:
1. Treadmill submaximal exercise test
2. Bicycle ergometer submaximal exercise test
3. Bench stepping submaximal exercise test
4. Other submaximal exercise test

Treadmill Submaximal Exercise Test

The test provides an estimate of functional aerobic VO_2 maximum. The VO_2 maximum has two-stage model:

Single stage model
To estimate the VO_2 maximum using the single stage model, use one submaximal heart rate and one workload. The submaximal heart rate ranges from 130 to 150 bpm. Men VO_2 maximum = SM VO_2 × $(HR_{max} - 61)/HR_{SM} - 61$
  Women VO_2 maximum = SM VO_2 × $(HR_{max} - 72)/HR_{SM} - 61$
  e.g., VO_2 for 40-year-old female
  Submaximal data stage 3

$VO_2 = 6.0$ MET (SM VO_2)
HR = 150 bpm (HR_{SM})
Max MR: 220 – age = HR_{SM}

Maximum heart rate equation is 220 minus Age. If the patients age is 45 years, then maximum heart rate is 175 BPM.

VO_{2max} = SM VO_2 × (HR_{max} – 72)/HR_{SM} – 72
= 6 × (175 – 72)/(150 – 72)
= 6 × 103/78
= 6 × 1.3205
= 7.92 MET

Single-stage treadmill walking test

The single-stage treadmill walking for estimating the VO_2 maximum.

Indications

Low-risk and healthy adults 20–59 years of age.

Protocol

Walking speed ranges from 2.0 to 4.5 mph or 53.6 to 120.6 m/min.

This depends on the client's age, gender, and the fitness level. Initially, the test should begin with 4-minute warm-up at 0% grade. The heart rate should be 50–70% of the age of the patient.

The test consists of brisk walking for 4 minutes at 5% grade record in the heart rate.

VO_2 maximum in mL/kg/min
$VO_{2\,max}$ = 15.1 + 21.8 (speed mph) – 0.327 (HR bpm)
= –0.263 (speed × age years) + 0.00504 (HR × age)
= +5.48 (gender where female = 0, male = 1).

Multistage model

When the patient completes submaximal exercise test twice, then the values are considered for calculating $VO_{2\,max}$. But if the patient is able to complete submaximal test three times then second and third test results are taken into consideration to calculate $VO_{2\,max}$. The data used is from stages 2 and 3 to estimate the $VO_{2\,max}$.

The estimation of the $VO_{2\,max}$ by heart rate and workload. The data is then taken two or more submaximal stages of the treadmill test. The patient's heart rate can be in between 115 and 150 bpm.

Slope (b) = Difference between two submaximal workloads SM/changes in the submaximal heart rate.

$B = (SM_2 - SM_1)/HR_1 - HR_2$

Submaximal data stage 2:
  $VO_{2\,max}$ = 20.5 mL/kg/min (SM_2)
  HR = 140 bpm (HR_2)
Submaximal data stage 1
  $VO_{2\,max}$ = 14.1 mL/kg/min (SM_2)
  HR = 120 bpm (HR_1)
Maximum HR: 220 − age = 182 bpm
Slope (b) = ($SM_2 − SM_1$)/($HR_2 − HR_1$)
B = 20.5 − 14.1/140 − 120
B = 6.4/20 = 0.32
$VO_{2\,max}$ = SM_2 + B ($HR_{max} − HR_2$)
      = 20.5 + (0.32 (182 − 140))
      = 20.5 + (0.32 × 42) = 20.5 + 13.44 = 33.94.

Bicycle Ergometer Submaximal Exercise Test

The protocol uses 3 or 4 consecutive 3-minute workload on the bicycle ergometer designed to raise the heart rate between 110 and 150 bpm. The pedal rate is 50 rpm and the initial workload is 150 kgm/min (25 W). If heart rate is <80 bpm, set the second workload at 750 kgm/min.

The rest are as follows:
First workload is 150 kgm. The heart rates are
HR < 80, HR = 80–90, HR = 90–100, HR > 100

Workload	HR < 80	HR = 80–90	HR = 90–100	HR > 100
Second	750 kgm	600 kgm	450 kgm	300 kgm
Third	900 kgm	750 kgm	600 kgm	450 kgm
Fourth	1,050 kgm	900 kgm	750 kgm	600 kgm

Calculate the energy expenditure (VO_2) for the last two workloads using the ACSM metabolic equation.

Bench Stepping Submaximal Test

The bench stepping submaximal test consists of two protocols, which are described in the following sections.

Astrand–Rhyming step test protocol

This protocol calculates $VO_{2\,max}$ from the post exercise heart rate during bench stepping. The patient number of steps are calculated in 5 minutes period. The height of the bench is 33 cm or 13 in. for women and 40 cm or 15.75 in. for men.

Measure the postexercise heart rate by counting the number of beats between 15 and 30 seconds after exercise (convert this 15-second count to beats per minute by multiplying by 4). The nomogram can be used for correct $VO_{2\,max}$ if the patient's age is 25 years less or more.

Queens Step Protocol
The female patient steps 22/min and male patient steps 24/min for 3 min. The height of the bench is 16–25 in. or 41.3 cm. After exercise, the patient will be standing, wait for 5 second, and take 15 second heart rate count. Cover the counts to beats per minute by multiplying by 4. If in group teach patient how to take their own pulse rate. Test $VO_{2\,max}$.

Other Submaximal Exercise Test

Stair climbing submaximal test protocols
This estimates the aerobic capacity. Two types of step ergometers are used. They are Stair Master 4000PT and Stair Master 6000 PT.

The 4,000 PT has step pedals that go up and down and 6,000 PT has revolving stair case.

Rowing ergometer submaximal step protocol
To know the patient $VO_{2\,max}$.

The patient will perform rowing exercise and note down the heart rate, distance, and duration.

Field tests
To measure the cardiovascular fitness of the larger group. This test is practical, inexpensive, less time-consuming, and easily administered. The test can be used for age-group of ≤40 years in males and women of ≤50 years. This will assess the cardiovascular endurance by walking, running, swimming, cycling or bench stepping, and measuring both the pre-exercise heart rate and postexercise heart rate.

Distance run tests
This is to evaluate the aerobic capacity. The individual should be able to run the given distance in less time or more distance in given time. The distance is of 1.0 or 1.5 mi (1,600–2,400).

For example, select 1.0 mi or 1,600 m or duration of 9-minute run and 1.0- or 1.5-mi runs.

Nine- or 12-minute run test
Nine- or 12-minute run test on a flat track.

Cardiac Rehabilitation

One- and 1.5-mi run/walk test
Conduct the 1.5-mi run/walk test on a 400-m track or flat odometer or measuring wheel to measure the distance. For 1.5 mi, patient should fastly cover the distance in the fastest time by running, walking includes covering the shortest distance in the short possible time.

One-mile jogging test
The patient should run as fast as possible and give their best effort. So submaximal 1-mi-track jogging test for 18–29-year-old women and men. The patient should be comfortable moderate jogging pace, postexercise heart rate. The time for 1 mi is 8 minutes for males and 9 minutes for females and postexercise heart rate not exceed 180 bpm. In 1-mi test 2- or 3-minute warm-up jog.

Walking test
To assess the cardiovascular fitness for males and females of 20–69 years. This is fast walking in the older or sedentary individual of about 1.0 mi at the earliest and check the heart rate. The walking course is flat, 400 m track. Stretch for 5–10 min before the test is taken. Ask the patient to wear the good walking shoes and loose-fitting clothes.

Step test
This test is to check the cardiovascular fitness. This is done for large groups and is inexpensive, useful for aerobic fitness, and pulse rate should be checked regularly.

Additional field test
The 12-minute cycling test use bike with three speeds conducted on hard and flat surface and wind velocity is <10 mph. The odometer is used to measure distance traveled in 12 minutes.

Twelve-minute swimming test
The patient can use any stroke and can take rest. This test is least preferred because the results of this test depends upon the skill of the patient.

Wait test
This is to assess the cardiorespiratory fitness in young children where the treadmill or the bicycle ergometer is used. The age-group will be of 5–17 years. 1.0-mi or run/walk test for 8–17 years and 0.5-mi run/wet test for 5–7 years.

GRADED EXERCISE TEST PROTOCOLS

1. The test should start with the warm-up for 3 or more minutes.
2. The initial exercise intensity should be about 2 or 3 MET.
3. Duration of the each work stage is for 3 minutes and also for the steady state of the patient.
4. The total test duration will be of 8–12 minutes.

Aerobic Capacity or Cardiorespiratory Fitness–Graded Exercise Testing

1. The GXT is done and $VO_{2\,max}$ is measured.
2. The maximum exercise testing is done or men >40 years and females >50 years.
3. Before, during, and after maximal and submaximal tests, check the heart rate, blood pressure, and resting pulse rate.
4. The common modes of the exercise testing are treadmill, bicycle ergometer, and bench stepping.
5. Field tests are done for the aerobic capacity and not for the diagnostic purpose.
6. For the cardiovascular fitness of the large groups, the distance run test, walking test, and step tests are used.
7. The distance run test is at least for 9 minutes for the aerobic functional assessment. The distance is 1–3 mi or 1,600–4,800 m or 9–12 minutes.

Advantages and Disadvantages

S. No.	Advantages	Disadvantages
1.	Natural form of exercise	Risk of accident
2.	Easy to calibrate	Patient will be anxious
3.	High $VO_{2\,max}$	Difficult to obtain

Exercise Prescription

1. Intensity: The stress test must be done before giving the exercise regime.
2. The exercises should begin with the low-level intensity.
3. The duration is about 15–60 minutes.
4. The frequency is about 3–5 days/week with 2 days of rest between the sessions.

MET level: The MET level is used to compare the energy costs of various activities and energy costs at rest.

Cardiac Rehabilitation

The following are the MET levels for the selected activities:

S. No.	MET level	Activity
1.	1.5–2	• Standing • Walking (1 mph) • Desk work • Sitting • Reading • Self-feeding • Extremities active-assisted exercises in supine lying or sitting
2.	2–3	• Walking (2 mph) • Bicycling (5 mph) • Typing • Standing • Performing the mat exercises • Lightweight moving of 2–3 lb
3.	3–4	• Walking (3 mph) • Cycling (6 mph) • Slow stair climbing • Balance • Mild resistance mat exercises
4.	4–5	• Walking (3.5 mph) • Cycling (8 mph)
5.	5–6	• Walking (4 mph) • Stairs/step aerobics
6.	6–7	• Cycling (11 mph) • Walking (5 mph)
7.	7–10	• Jogging • Cycling (13 mph) • Walking (5.5 mph)
8.	11–12	• Climbing hill • Running (5 minute mile)
9.	13–14	• Running 7 minute mile

Risk Factors

The risk factors commonly seen with the patient suffering from the cardiovascular problem are:
1. Smoking
2. Hypertension
3. Elevated cholesterol level
4. Age
5. Diabetes
6. Sedentary lifestyle
7. Family history
8. Male gender

Guidelines for the Management of the Risk Factors

1. Lipid management
2. Hypertension management
3. Diabetic management
4. Smoking cessation
5. Weight management
6. Psychological management

S. No.	Management	Evaluate	Aim	Plan
1.	Lipid	Check the total cholesterol, HDL, LDL, and triglycerides	• LDL < 100 mg/dL or if more • HDL > 40 mg/dL or more	• Nutritional counseling • Weight management • Exercise • Smoking cessation
2.	Hypertension	Check blood pressure	• If BP < 140/90 mm Hg Systolic BP > 130 mm Hg Diastolic BP > 85 mm Hg • If BP = 130/85 mm Hg Systolic BP > 140 mm Hg Diastolic BP > 90 mm Hg	• Exercise weight management, sodium restriction, alcohol and smoking cessation • All of the above and lifestyle modification
3.	Diabetes	Fasting blood glucose and in diabetics HbA1C	Fasting blood glucose <110 mg/dL HbA1C < 7 Hypoglycemic therapy	• Weight reduction • Exercise • Oral hypoglycemic agents or insulin. Before and after exercise monitor the blood glucose level. Train the patient to check the postexercise hypoglycemia. If blood glucose is >300 mL/dL, discourage the exercise
4.	Smoking	Enquire about the smoking habits, amount, and duration of smoking	Complete cessation is encouraged	• Education • Counseling • Drug therapy

Contd...

Contd...

S. No.	Management	Evaluate	Aim	Plan
5.	Weight	BMI—weight, height, and waist circumference	BMI should be in between 21 and 25 kg/m^2	Total calorie intake should be reduced and the energy expenditure should be increased by regular diet and exercise
6.	Psychological	Anger, anxiety, depression, and distress	Stress management	Counseling, education, and treatment by the mental health professional

Pulmonary Rehabilitation 9

INTRODUCTION

The pulmonary rehabilitation is a multidisciplinary program of a patient with acute and chronic respiratory diseases that are designed to increase the overall quality of life of the patient. Pulmonary rehabilitation is for the patients who are diagnosed with respiratory ailments or pulmonary diseases.

INDICATIONS

1. Chronic respiratory failure
2. Chronic obstructive pulmonary diseases (COPDs) such as asthma, bronchitis, bronchiectasis, and cystic fibrosis
3. Reduced capacity to perform daily life activities
4. Dyspnea
5. Surgical intervention

CONTRAINDICATIONS

1. Pulmonary hypertension
2. Ischemic heart disease
3. Liver dysfunction
4. Cancer
5. Renal failure

EFFECTS AND USES

1. Pulmonary rehabilitation will help the patient for management and maintenance of the disease by continuing physical therapy pulmonary rehabilitation program designed according to the condition.
2. Improves the quality of the life and helps to maintain healthy lifestyle.
3. Decreases anxiety and depression and helps to overcome by using relaxation techniques.
4. Asthma patients have to be deal with the sports and weather precautions and care to be taken and focus on breathing pattern.

Pulmonary Rehabilitation

5. Pulmonary rehabilitation decreases the period of hospitalization by following special designed maintenance program.
6. Pulmonary rehabilitation program also helps in good understanding about the medication and its side effects and also encourages to carry the emergency medication always.

GOALS

1. To decrease disability
2. To reduce symptoms
3. To increase physical activity
4. To improve quality of life.

The pulmonary rehabilitation program is basically divided into four phases. They are:
1. Inpatient phase
2. Outpatient phase
3. Self care program phase
4. Self-monitoring and maintenance phase.

Inpatient Phase

1. The patient will be referred by the doctors. Patient is either in hospital or skilled nursing facility. The resident will be assessed by the physical therapist, occupational therapist and speech therapist. Based on the assessment the patient is put on the therapy for the duration of 3 to 5 days a week for 6 to 8 weeks depending on the patient diagnosis and requirement of rehabilitation services. The resident is put on pulmonary rehabilitation program.
2. During this phase, the patient performs exercises to improve strength, endurance, and flexibility, and also breathing techniques are taught.
3. Techniques for energy conservation, functional activity tolerance, activity pacing, relaxation techniques to decrease anxiety and shortness of breath and reducing complications are performed.
4. The patient is taught bed mobility activities like rolling to the both sides using handrails, supine to sit, sitting at the edge of the bed. All these activities help the patient to get out of the bed and avoid staying in the bed to prevent bed rest complications.
5. Teach the techniques to clear unwanted secretions of lung by teaching breathing exercises and coughing techniques.
6. Teaching the patient and also training of family members are performed about home exercise program.

7. The patient depending on the diagnosis the discharge planning is planned by the social worker and rehabilitation group work towards the goals in achieving using any assistive devices or adaptive devices.

Outpatient Phase

This phase is divided into three phases.

Education and Management Phase

1. This phase includes training and education about cessation of smoking, weight management, proper usage of medication, and management of condition.
2. Aerobic exercises such as strengthening and endurance exercises.
3. Assessment of exercise tolerance by teaching self-monitoring of vitals such as blood pressure, O_2 saturation, and heart rate.
4. Breathing exercises.
5. Proper usage of pulmonary devices such as acapella, peak flow meters, and nebulizers.

Self-care Program Phase

The patient is educated about the pulmonary conditions, their risk factors, modifications, exercise program, medications, their side effects and emergency medications to be carried at all time and use them during the emergency situation.

Self-monitoring and Maintenance Phase

The patient is well trained with self-monitoring of vital signs like using pulse oximeter for oxygen saturation and pulse rate, blood pressure apparatus for blood pressure, heart rate. The patient should also know their upper and lower limit readings and care to be taken when symptoms are developed.

THE OVERALL PLAN AND TREATMENT OF PULMONARY REHABILITATION

S. No.	Aims	Plans
1.	To loosen the secretions	Massage manipulations, breathing exercises, postural drainage, and inhalation therapy
2.	To aid in removal of secretions	Coughing, huffing, forced expiratory technique, and suction

Contd...

Contd...

S. No.	Aims	Plans
3.	To induce relaxation	Relaxation technique is demonstrated
4.	To teach breathing control	Breathing control techniques are taught
5.	To prevent postural deformity	Teach postural awareness
6.	To maintain the mobility of the upper extremity, lower extremity, and trunk	Mobility exercises of the upper limb, lower limb and trunk
7.	To give home advice	Home care management for preventing of recurrence of the symptoms

ASSESSMENT FOR PULMONARY REHABILITATION

1. Patient history
2. Physical examination
3. Previous history
4. Exercise capacity and endurance
5. Mini-mental state examination (MMSE) and neurobehavioral cognitive status examination (NCSE), age, and hypoxemia
6. Emotional disturbance, depression, and anxiousness
7. Nutritional assessment
8. Body weight and body composition are measured using body mass index (BMI) chart.

OUTCOME ASSESSMENT

Impairment

The impairment can be defined as is the loss of function resulting from disease.

Diagnosis of impairment can be done by two tests as described in the following subsections.

Force Expiratory Volume

The forced expiratory volume can be defined as volume of the air expired forcibly after maximum inspiration in a second is forced expiratory volume (FEV).

FEV_1: The volume of air expired forcibly after maximum inspiration in one second is FEV_1.

Forced vital capacity: This is the maximum volume of air expired forcibly after maximum inspiration.

In a healthy person: FEV1/FVC = 80%

Vital capacity: It is the maximum volume of the air expired after maximum inspiration.
VC = 4,000 mL or 4 L

The values of VC, FEV1, and its percentage are measured by Vitalograph spirometer. Some of them are:

S. No.	Condition	VC	FEV1	FVC/VC	Example
1.	Normal person	4 L	3.2 L	80%	–
2.	Obstructive airway disease	3.2	1.3	41%	Chronic bronchitis, asthma, emphysema
3.	Restrictive airway disease	2	1.6	80%	Pneumonia ankylosing spondylitis

Pulmonary Function Tests

The pulmonary function tests are the diagnostic test performed to know how well the lungs are functioning. The pulmonary function test also gives information about diagnosis and treatment to be given for specific lung disorders.

Indications:
- To measure the lung volume
- To measure the lung capacity
- To measure the flow rates
- To measure the gas exchange
- To measure the diffusion capacity
- To measure inspiratory and expiratory pressure
- To measure blood gas levels.

The following are the lung volumes, lung capacities and flow rate:

Lung volumes

The following are the lung volumes described:
- **Tidal volume:** The volume of the air breathed in and out in a single normal quiet respiration is called tidal volume. It is about 500 mL.
- **Inspiratory reserve volume:** The additional amount of the air inspired forcefully after the end of the normal inspiration is called inspiratory reserved volume. It is about 3,300 mL or 3.3 L.
- **Expiratory reserve volume:** The additional amount of the air that can be expired out forcefully after normal expiration is called expiratory reserve volume. The normal value is 1,000 mL or 1 L.
- **Residual volume:** The amount of the air remaining in the lung even after the forced expiration is called residual volume. The normal value is 1,200 mL or 1.2 L.

The important facts about residual volume are:
1. Residual volume maintains the contour of the lung.
2. Residual volume helps to aerate the blood in between breathing and during expiration.

Lung capacities
The lung capacities include two or more primary volumes. They are:
1. *Inspiratory capacity:* This is the maximum volume of air that can be inspired starting from the end expiratory position. Its value is 3,800 mL (IC = TV + IRV = 500 + 3,300 = 3,800).
2. *Vital capacity:* This is the maximum amount of the air that can be expelled out forcefully after a maximal deep inspiration. Its value is 4,800 mL (VC = IRV + TV + ERV = 3,300 + 500 + 1,000 = 4,800 mL).
3. *Functional residual capacity:* This is the volume of the air remaining in the lungs after normal expiration. Its value is 2,200 mL (FRC + ERV + RV = 1,000 + 1,200 = 2,200 mL).
4. *Total lung capacity:* This is the amount of the air present in the lungs after a deep inspiration. It includes all the volumes. Its value is TLC = IRV + TV + ERV + RV = 3,300 + 500 + 1,000 + 1,200 = 6,000 mL.

Forced expiratory flow rate:
A peak flow meter provides a quick and simple indication of airway obstruction. The test is performed three times with rest in between the test. The results considered are best result of three tests performed.

Suggestions to the Patient

1. The patient is asked to avoid tight clothes.
2. Avoid heavy meal.
3. The patient is asked to quit smoking. The patient is explained about the procedure of the test to be performed.
4. If the first reading is taken in one position then other two should also be taken in the same position.
5. The physical therapist should demonstrate the technique with mouthpiece.
6. The patient should hold the mouthpiece tightly.
7. The patient is asked to take a deep breath till the lungs feel full then blow out air short and sharp.

Aim

1. This is very important for patients with unstable asthma because lung function can decline to 50 or 60% of normal before symptoms are noticeable.

2. This is useful in the chronic asthma to determine the right drug.
3. To evaluate ventilation by assessing the factors affecting the movement of gas in and out of the lungs.
4. To guide the diagnosis, treatment plan, and prognosis.
5. To help therapist to plan for therapeutic goals, appropriate intervention to the pulmonary problems, and identify the permanent respiratory impairment.

Guidelines

1. The pulmonary function test evaluates airway responsivity, ventilatory regulation, and ventilatory mechanics.
2. The pulmonary function tests allow the effect of hypoxia and hypercapnia.
3. The pulmonary function tests help in the assessment of ventilatory mechanics which is the measurement of lung volumes occur in restrictive diseases like pneumonia, intestinal lung disease, pleural effusion, pleurisy, pneumonia, and forced flow rates decreases in obstructive disease such as chronic bronchitis, emphysema, asthma, bronchiectasis, and cystic fibrosis.
4. The assessment of the ventilatory mechanics also permits evaluation of the effectiveness of therapy.
5. The pulmonary function tests helps to find out the general progress of the disease process.
6. The pulmonary function tests helps in the determination of the pulmonary impairment.

Tests Performed by the Physical Therapist

A rough estimation of the airway obstruction can be made by asking the patient to blow out a lighted match held 6 in. from the mouth, failure to do so suggest an FEV1 of < 1 L.

▌MEASUREMENT OF THE PULMONARY FUNCTION

1. Spirometer
2. Gas transfer tests
3. Exercise testing
4. Quantitative perfusion/ventilation scanning
5. Six-minute walk
6. Stair climbing

Spirometer

The method by which the lung volumes and capacities are measured is called spirometry. The simple instrument used for this purpose is called spirometer. The modified spirometer is known as respirometer.

The spirometer can be used only for a single breath. The repeated cycles of respiration cannot be recorded by using the spirometer because the carbon dioxide accumulated in the spirometer cannot be removed and oxygen or fresh air cannot be provided to the subject.

Respirometer

This is the modified spirometer. This has the facility of removing the carbon dioxide and supply the oxygen. The carbon dioxide is removed by placing soda lime inside the instrument. The oxygen is supplied to the instrument from the oxygen cylinder by a suitable valve system.

Spirogram

The record of the lung volumes and capacities using spirometer or respirometer is called spirogram. The downward deflection of the spirogram indicates expiration and the upward curve denotes inspiration.

Computerized Spirometer

This is a solid-state electronic equipment. The subject has to respire into a sophisticated transducer, which is connected to the instrument by means of a cable.

The residual volume, functional residual capacity, and the total lung capacity are measured by the nitrogen washout technique and helium dilution technique, not with the spirometry.

Helium Dilution Technique

Functional residual capacity

The respirometer is filled with the air containing a known quantity of helium. Initially, the subject breathes normally, then after the end of the expiration, the subject breathes from the respirometer. The helium from the respirometer enters the lungs and starts mixing with the air in the lungs. After few minutes of breathing, the concentration of helium in the respirometer becomes equal to the concentration of helium in the lungs of the subject. This is called the equilibrium of helium. The concentration of helium in respirometer is determined.

$FRC = V(C_1 - C_2)/C_2$

C_1 is the initial concentration of helium in the respirometer, C_2 is the final concentration of the helium in the respirometer, and V is the initial volume of air in the respirometer.

Example: V = 5,000 mL, C_1 = 15%, C_2 = 10%
FRC = 5,000 (15/100 – 10/100) mL divided by 10/1,000 = 2,500 mL

Residual volume
The subject should start breathing from the respirometer after forced expiration.

Nitrogen Washout Method

The concentration of nitrogen in the air is 80%. The total quantity of nitrogen in the lungs is measured so that the amount of air in the lungs can be calculated.

Functional residual capacity
The subject is asked to breathe normally. After the end of the normal expiration, the subject inspires pure oxygen through a valve and expires into a Douglas bag. This procedure is repeated for 6–7 minutes till the nitrogen in lungs is displaced by oxygen. The nitrogen comes to the Douglas bag.

The FRC is calculated as:
1. Volume of air collected in Douglas bag
2. Concentration of nitrogen in the Douglas bag FRC = C_1 multiply V/C_2

V = Volume of air collected = 40,000 mL
C_1 = Concentration of nitrogen in the collected air = 50%
C_2 = Normal concentration of nitrogen in the air = 80% FRC = 2,500 mL.

Residual volume
The subject starts inhaling pure oxygen after the end of the forceful expiration.

Gas Transfer Tests

Arterial blood gases may be used to evaluate gas transfer and ventilation. The partial pressure of carbon dioxide provides the useful information of the alveolar ventilation. There is a minimum alteration that indicates severe dysfunction of gas exchange.

Exercise Testing

Measurement of exercise capacity evaluates the combined performance of cardiac and respiratory system. The maximum uptake is preoperative outcome and used to identify surgical requirement for the patients.

Quantitative Perfusion/Ventilation Scanning

Radionuclide lung perfusion/ventilation scanning estimates the contribution of each lung, regions and lung function. It is used to predict pulmonary function after resection, pneumonectomy, and lobectomy.

Six-minute Walk

This is an inexpensive, easily performed test. It is for the chronic obstructive lung disease, preoperative evaluation of the thoracic surgery patient.

Procedure

The patient is instructed to walk on a predetermined course as far and as fast as possible. The distance will be over 1,000 feet. This is for uncomplicated postoperative recovery.

Stair Climbing

This is an exercise tolerance test done by climbing upstairs.

Clinical Application

1. Preoperative evaluation
2. Diagnosis of the functional pulmonary disorders
3. Obstructive ventilatory disorders such as chronic bronchitis, emphysema, asthma cystic fibrosis bronchiectasis
4. Restrictive ventilatory disorders such as fibrosing alveolitis, interstitial pneumonitis, and sarcoidosis and chest wall deformities

DISABILITY

This is the inability to perform an activity due to the lung disease. The diagnosis of the disability is done based on the following subsections.

Field Test

This test is for the larger groups.

Uses of This Test

1. This test is practical
2. The test is inexpensive
3. The test consumes less time

4. The test can use to classify cardiorespiratory fitness of healthy men below or equal to 40 years and women less than or equal to 50 years.

Contraindications of the Test

The patient with coronary artery disease cannot take this test because electrocardiogram and blood pressure cannot be monitored.

Effects and Uses

This test helps to assess cardiorespiratory endurance of the patient by asking the patient to perform walking, running, swimming and cycling.

Technique

This test measures post exercise heart rate.

Handicap

The inability to perform an activity because of impairment and disability.

Diagnosis: Tred walk test: This is the test developed by Mr Tred.

Aim

To assess cardiovascular fitness of both the sexes of ages between 20 and 69 years.

Uses

1. Can assess older age group
2. Useful for sedentary individuals

Guidelines

The individual should wear good walking shoes and clothing should be loose.

Method

Fast walking of about 1.0 mi. This gives submaximal VO_2.

Technique

The individual should walk 1.0 mi as quickly as possible, and at the end of the test, the heart rate is checked by continuing the pulse for 15 seconds.

The walking tract should be flat with no interruptions in its way and the length of the tract should be 400 m. The individual can do stretching for 5-10 minutes to locate the walking time and check postexercise heart rate (beats per minute) on the appropriate chart for the client age and gender.

The chart is based on the body weight.
Women: 125 lb or 56.8 kg
Men: 170 lb or 77.3 kg

If the individual weight is more than this, then the overestimation of cardiovascular fitness occurs.

PULMONARY REHABILITATION PROGRAM– RESPIRATORY CARE

1. To aid in loosening of the secretions: The following techniques are used to loosen the secretions. They are:
   a. Massage manipulations
   b. Breathing exercises
   c. Postural drainage
   d. Inhalation therapy
   e. Humidification
   f. Intermittent positive pressure breathing
2. To remove the secretions
   a. Effective coughing
   b. Huffing
   c. Forced expiration technique
   d. Suction
3. To induce relaxation
4. To enhance breathing control
5. To bring awareness of posture
6. To mobilize upper extremity, lower extremity, and trunk
7. To teach home management

   Massage manipulations: Massage is the scientific manipulation of the soft tissues of body done with the palmar aspect of hands or fingers.

Type of Manipulations

The types of manipulations used are:
1. Clapping
2. Vibration
3. Shaking

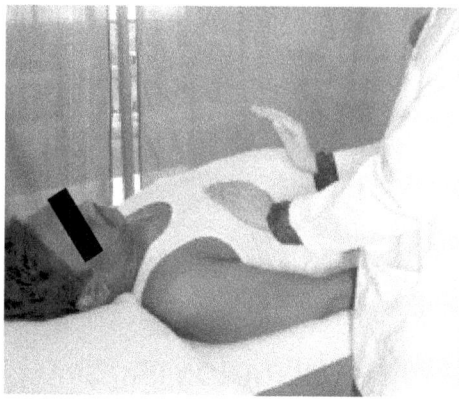

Fig. 9.1: Clapping.

Clapping

The clapping technique is done with hands cupped position that strike the chest wall one after the other **(Fig. 9.1)**.

Position of the patient
Prone lying with blanket over chest.

Position of the therapist
The therapist is in stride standing position. Arms are kept at 30° abduction, elbow flexed to 90°, hands are cupped and finger and thumb are adducted, metatarsophalangeal joint of index and middle and ring fingers are slightly flexed.

Technique
There is a rapid control of the flexion and extension at the wrist.

Indication
Chronic respiratory disorders.

Vibration

The vibration manipulation of the distal part of upper limb is used to transmit the mechanical energy to the body. Vibrations are produced in hands and fingers.

Types
1. Vibration
2. Shaking

The vibration technique is performed by placing the hands in both upward and downward direction with forearm in full

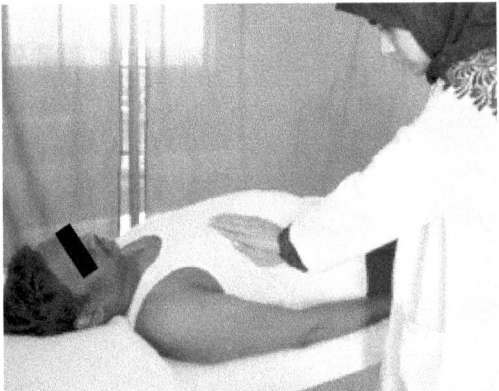

Fig. 9.2: Vibration.

pronation, wrist dorsiflexion to 70–90 degrees, hands in contact with the patient's skin **(Fig. 9.2)**.

Shaking forearm in mid prone position, the wrist held in 0–10 angle of dorsiflexion. The hand moves in medial-lateral direction.

Technique

The therapist is in walk standing position. The elbow extended and shoulder little flexed. One hand is placed over the other which remains in contact with the chest wall of the patient.

Transfer the body weight of the therapist to patient chest through extended upper extremity and tenses up arm, shoulder muscle. This causes oscillatory movement of hand in upward and downward direction and transmits mechanical energy to patient chest.

Vibration is performed during expiratory phase of the respiration. The patient is asked to inhale deeply and then blow out all air through mouth.

Vibration is initiated just before the expiratory phase and extended to the beginning of inspiratory phase. Manual vibration gives frequency of 20 Hz. Contraction of upper limb muscle vibration can also produce in fingertips or single palm.

Physiological uses
1. Dislodge thick sputum from bronchial wall
2. Mobilizes secretions

Shaking

The shaking transmits oscillatory mechanical energy to the chest wall **(Fig. 9.3)**. The shaking oscillation are produced in the sideway direction using radial and ulnar deviation occurring at the wrist joint.

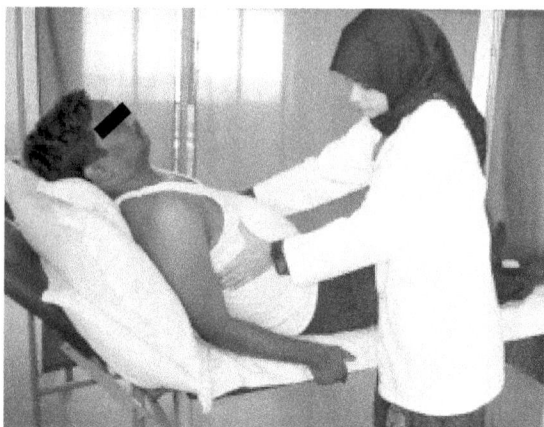

Fig. 9.3: Shaking.

Technique

The position of the therapist is walk standing position and therapist at both hands are positioned over the affected lobe of the patient's chest wall. The shoulder is adducted elbow slightly flexed.

Position of the patient

Position 1

The patient is in supine lying. The therapist places both the hands on each side of the anterior chest wall.

The other position of the hands are; one hand on the anterior aspect and the other hand on the posterior aspect of the chest wall on the same side.

Position 2

The patient is in side-lying position. The hand placement either can be using both the hands on the upper lateral chest wall or one hand on the anterior chest wall and other hand on the posterior chest wall on the same side of the upper chest.

Shaking is done only during the expiration phase. The therapist transfers the body weight to the patient chest and produces upward and downward movement of upper extremity. This gives vigorous shaking to the chest wall.

Uses

1. Dislodge secretions from the bronchial tree.
2. The sputum is shifted from smaller to the larger bronchioles.
3. The shaking over the sternum during the respiration stimulates the cough reflex.

Contraindications
1. Hemoptysis
2. Pleuritic pain
3. Pulmonary tuberculosis
4. Rib fractures
5. Osteoporosis

BREATHING EXERCISES

The breathing exercises are useful to loosen the secretions.

Aims

1. To strengthen the muscles of respiration
2. To improve ventilation
3. To improve oxygenation
4. To improve gas exchange
5. To lessen the work of the breathing
6. To teach active range of motion exercises to the shoulder and trunk that help to expand the chest
7. To facilitate deep breathing
8. To stimulate the cough reflex
9. To improve pulmonary status
10. To improve patients overall endurance
11. To improve the function of activities of daily living
12. To promote relaxation
13. To prevent pulmonary impairment
14. To improve patients overall functional capacity
15. To deal with shortness of breath attack
16. To improve strength and co-ordination of respiratory muscles

The breathing exercises are often combined with the postural drainage, exercises, respiratory therapy devices, and medications.

Indications

1. Pre- and postoperative cardiac surgery conditions
2. Acute lung diseases
3. Chronic lung conditions
4. Spinal cord injury
5. Muscular dystrophy
6. Kyphosis
7. Scoliosis
8. Stress management
9. Relaxation

Principles

1. The instruction to the patient regarding the therapy should be given clearly and in simple manner.
2. The treatment area should be quiet.
3. Explain the patient the importance of breathing exercise.
4. Patient should be comfortable and relaxed.
5. Patient should wear loose clothing and avoid restrictive clothing.
6. Position of the patient is crook lying in bed with head and trunk elevated 45°.
7. Abdominal muscles are relaxed when head and trunk are well supported, flexing the hips and knees and legs are supported with a pillow.
8. As the patient is perfect in this position, progression is taught in other position such as supine lying, sitting, and standing positions.
9. The patient is taught relaxation techniques.
10. Patient should practice on his own and should be perfect with the correct technique.

Precautions

1. The expiration should be relaxed and passive.
2. Never encourage the patient to expire forcibly as this causes increased airway resistance and bronchospasm.
3. The patient should not prolong expire as this mixed with the next inspiration; therefore breathing pattern becomes irregular and inefficient.
4. The patient should not use accessory muscles and upper chest to initiate inspiration.
5. To avoid hyperventilation, the patient should practice deep breathing for 3-4 times inspiration and expiration.

Classification

The breathing exercises are classified into:
1. Diaphragmatic breathing
2. Segmental breathing
   a. Apical breathing
   b. Lateral costal breathing
   c. Posterior basal breathing
   d. Lingular breathing
3. Ventilatory muscle training
   a. Diaphragmatic training using weights

b. Inspiratory resistance training
   c. Incentive respiratory spirometry
4. Glossopharyngeal breathing
5. Pursed lip breathing

Diaphragmatic Breathing

Aims
1. To improve gas exchange
2. To improve oxygenation
3. To improve ventilation
4. To improve ascent or descent of the diaphragm
5. To mobilize lung secretion during postural drainage
6. To decrease work of the breathing

Procedure

Position of the patient: Half lying supported by the pillows.

Position of the therapist: The physiotherapist stands beside the patient.

Technique **(Figs. 9.4 and 9.5)**: The hands should be placed on the rectus abdominis below the anterior costal margin. Initially, the therapist places the hands on the patient abdomen and asks the patient to inspire so that the abdomen bulges out and contracts and when the patient expires the abdomen falls back to normal position. Ask the patient to breathe in through the nose and breathe out through the mouth. Practice the same 3 or 4 times then rest for a brief period of time. Initially, the physical therapist demonstrates the technique then trains the patient to practice the same on his own by keeping hands on the abdomen and during expiration feels the contraction of the abdominals.

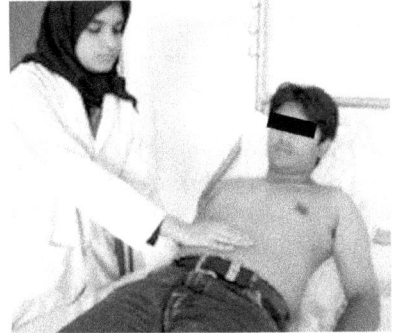

Fig. 9.4: Diaphragmatic breathing.

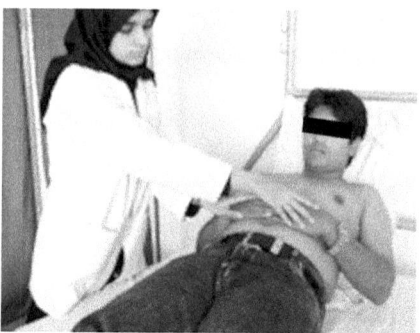

Fig. 9.5: Training the patient to perform the diaphragmatic breathing.

Segmental Breathing

Indication: Hypoventilation is also called respiratory depression where there is insufficient ventilation for the gas exchange to occur resulting in respiratory acidosis and hypercapnia (increased carbon dioxide concentration). It leads to respiratory arrest, breathing stops and causes death. The underlying condition is treated first and if the patient is obese the patient should work on loosing weight and bi-level positive airway pressure (BIPAP—these are small masks placed on nose and mouth and patient is supplied by oxygen during sleep to prevent sleep apnea). But when the patient is awake the therapist trains the patient using segmental breathing where patient is taught to expand the localized areas of the lungs while the other areas of lung remain quiet. This technique prevents hypoventilation of the lungs.

The second type of breathing is apical breathing

Indications: Lobectomy.

Position of the patient: Sitting.

Position of the physiotherapist: The therapist stands in front of the patient and applies the pressure below the clavicle with the fingertips.

Unilateral apical breathing

During inspiration: The physiotherapist applies the stretch downward and inward to the chest and muscle moves in the direction of outward and upward **(Figs. 9.6 to 9.8)**. This stretches the external intercostal muscle on the side of the pressure, i.e., right side or left side.

During expiration: The physiotherapist with palms gives firm downward pressure, and the ribcage is moved downward and inward on the side of the pressure, i.e., right side or left side.

Pulmonary Rehabilitation

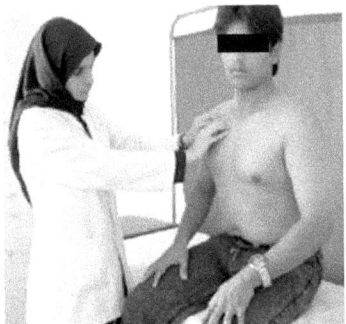

Fig. 9.6: Left unilateral apical breathing.

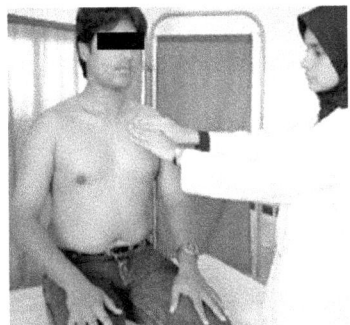

Fig. 9.7: Right unilateral apical breathing.

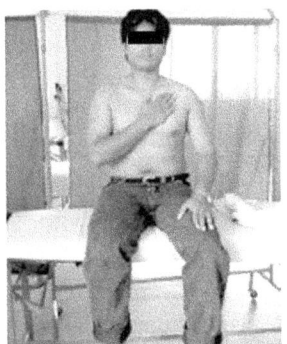

Fig. 9.8: Self-apical breathing.

Bilateral apical breathing

During inspiration: The physiotherapist applies the stretch downward and inward to the chest and muscle moves in the direction of outward and upward **(Fig. 9.9)**. This stretches the external intercostal muscle on the side of the pressure bilaterally.

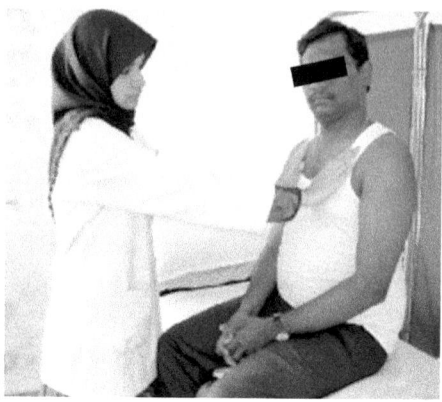

Fig. 9.9: Bilateral apical breathing.

During expiration: The physiotherapist with palms gives firm downward pressure, and the ribcage is moved downward and inward on the side of the pressure bilaterally.

Lateral costal breathing
This is also called lateral basal expansion.

The lateral coastal breathing is of two types. They are unilateral costal breathing and bilateral costal breathing.
- *Unilateral breathing:* Right or left side.
- *Position of the patient:* Crook lying.
- *Position of the therapist:* The physiotherapist should stand behind the patient and the hand is placed on the right side if right lateral costal breathing or on the left side if left lateral costal breathing.
- *Technique:* The chest moves upward and outward during inspiration and downward and inward during expiration.

Unilateral costal breathing

During inspiration: The physiotherapist applies the stretch downward and inward to the chest and muscle moves in the direction of outward and upward. This stretches the external intercostal muscle on the side of the pressure, i.e., right side or left side **(Fig. 9.10)**.

During expiration: The physiotherapist with palms gives firm downward pressure, and the ribcage is moved downward and inward on the side of the pressure, i.e., right side or left side.

Bilateral costal breathing
The physical therapist places both the hands on the bilateral aspect of the chest wall and the firm pressure is given for inspiration and expiration in the following direction **(Figs. 9.11 and 9.12)**.

Pulmonary Rehabilitation

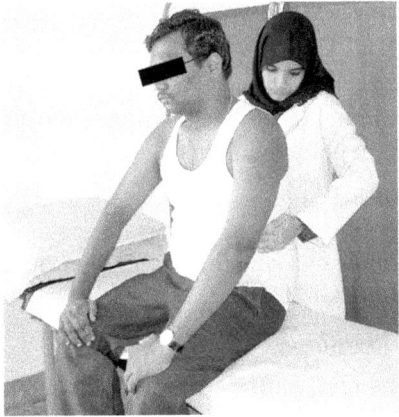

Fig. 9.10: Unilateral costal breathing.

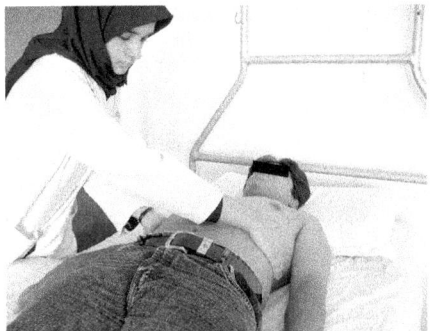

Fig. 9.11: Bilateral costal breathing in supine position.

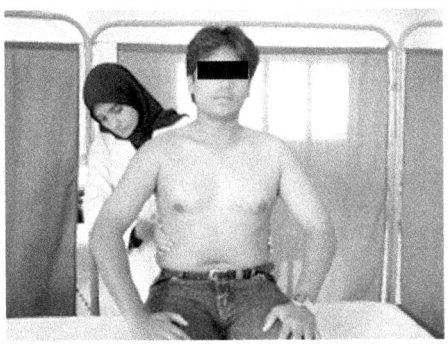

Fig. 9.12: Bilateral costal breathing in sitting position.

During inspiration: The physical therapist applies the stretch downward and inward to the chest and muscle moves in the direction of outward and upward. This stretches the external intercostal muscle on the side of the pressure bilaterally.

During expiration: The physical therapist with palms gives firm downward pressure, and the ribcage is moved downward and inward on the side of the pressure bilaterally.

Self-costal breathing

The patient is trained to perform the costal breathing unilaterally with hands and bilaterally by using the belt to perform independently at home, etc. **(Figs. 9.13 to 9.15)**.

Posterior basal breathing

Position of the patient: Sitting position and leaning forward on a pillow.

Position of the physiotherapist: The physiotherapist stands behind the patient and the therapist hands are on the posterior aspect of the lower ribs.

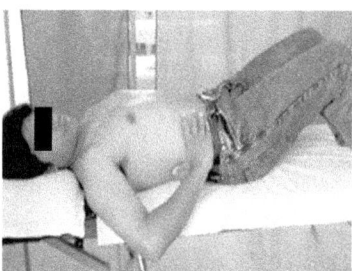

Fig. 9.13: Self-bilateral costal expansion.

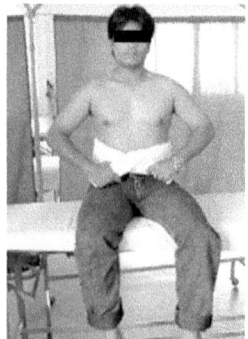

Fig. 9.14: Belt exercises for lateral costal breathing, applying resistance during inspiration.

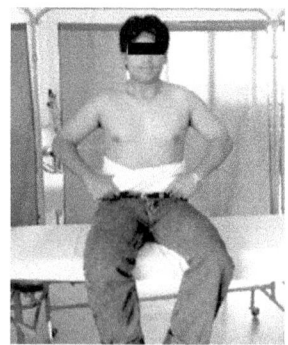

Fig. 9.15: Belt exercises for lateral costal breathing, applying assistance with pressure during expiration along the rib cage.

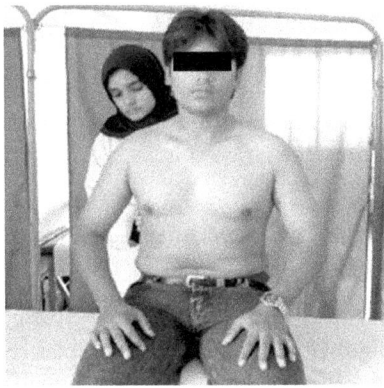

Fig. 9.16: Unilateral posterior basal breathing.

Procedure

Unilateral posterior basal breathing

During inspiration: The physiotherapist applies the stretch downward and inward to the chest and muscle moves in the direction of outward and upward. This stretches the external intercostal muscle on the side of the pressure, i.e., right side or left side **(Fig. 9.16)**.

During expiration: The physiotherapist with palms gives firm downward pressure, and the ribcage is moved downward and inward on the side of the pressure, i.e., right side or left side.

Bilateral posterior basal breathing

The physiotherapist places both the hands on the bilateral posterior aspect of the lower ribs of the chest wall, and the firm pressure is given for inspiration and expiration in the following direction **(Fig. 9.17)**.

During inspiration: The physiotherapist applies the stretch downward and inward to the chest and muscle moves in the direction of

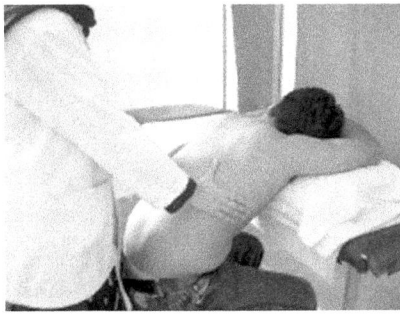

Fig. 9.17: Bilateral posterior basal breathing.

outward and upward. This stretches the external intercostal muscle on the side of the pressure bilaterally.

During expiration: The physiotherapist with palms gives firm downward pressure, and the ribcage is moved downward and inward on the side of the pressure bilaterally.

Lingular breathing

This is also called right middle lobe expansion as left lung has only two lobes **(Fig. 9.18)**.

Position of the patient: The patient is in sitting position.

Position of the physical therapist: The therapist stands behind the patient, and the hand is placed on the right side of the patient chest below the axilla.

Procedure
- *During inspiration:* The physical therapist applies the stretch downward and inward to the chest and muscle moves in the direction of outward and upward. This stretches the external intercostal muscle on the side of the pressure, i.e., right side.
- *During expiration:* The physical therapist with palms gives firm downward pressure, and the ribcage is moved downward and inward on the side of the pressure, i.e., right side.

Ventilatory Muscle Training

This technique is for improving the strength of the breathing muscle especially muscles of inspiration.

Indications
1. Acute pulmonary disease
2. Chronic pulmonary disease

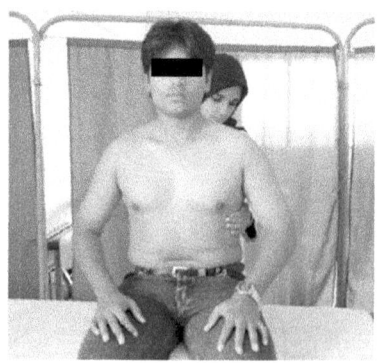

Fig. 9.18: Lingular breathing.

3. Weakness
4. Atrophy
5. Inefficiency of the muscles of the inspiration such as diaphragm and external intercostal

Types
The types of ventilator muscle training are:

Diaphragmatic training using weights
- *Position of the patient:* Supine lying
- *Procedure:* Put a small weight of about 3-5 lb over the epigastric region of the patient's abdomen. Ask the patient to breathe in against the resistance of the weight. Increase the number of times of the resistance breathing. The weight can be increased gradually and also the time duration can be increased for about 15 minutes. This strengthens the diaphragm. This is useful for the patient with weakness.

Inspiratory resistance training
This method increases the strength and endurance of the inspiratory muscle and decreases inspiratory muscle fatigue. This is through the breathing device called resistor. The resistor is put in the patient mouth and the patient inhales through the device, which gives resistance to the inspiratory muscles. The more narrow is the diameter of the airway, the more is the resistance. The time should be gradually increased to 20 to 30 minutes duration. Once strength and endurance are increased, the diameter of the tube is decreased.

Incentive respiratory spirometry
This is also called sustained maximal inspiratory maneuver.

Indication
1. Postoperative conditions
2. Neuromuscular disorders

Position of the patient: Supine lying

Procedure: The patient is asked to inspire the air 3-4 times slowly and exhales with the 4th breathe. Then put the spirometer into the mouth and ask the patient to inhale the air and hold for few seconds. This can be repeated 5-10 times a day.

Glossopharyngeal Breathing

Indication
1. Severe weakness of the inspiratory muscles

2. Spinal cord injuries
3. Postpolio patients with inspiratory muscle weakness

Aim
1. To increase patient inspiratory capacity
2. To prepare the patient for coughing
3. To advise the patient who has difficulty to breath so can use this technique.

Technique: The patient is asked to take gulps of air. The mouth is closed and the tongue moves the air to pharynx, the glottis gets opened and the air goes to the lungs. This way inspiration is increased and also the vital capacity of the lung.

Pursed Lip Breathing

Indication: COPDs such as chronic bronchitis, asthma, bronchiectasis, cystic fibrosis, and bronchitis **(Fig. 9.19)**.

Position of the patient: Patient in the comfortable and relaxed position

Technique: The physiotherapist places the hand on the abdominal muscle and the patient is asked to take a deep inspiration and with the lips pursed patient is asked to expire the air. The procedure is repeated many times with frequent relaxation periods in between.

Self-pursed lip breathing: The patient should practice the technique so that he can perform the technique independently. The technique is as follows.

The patient should place the hands on the abdomen and take a deep inspiration and with the lips pursed expire the air. The

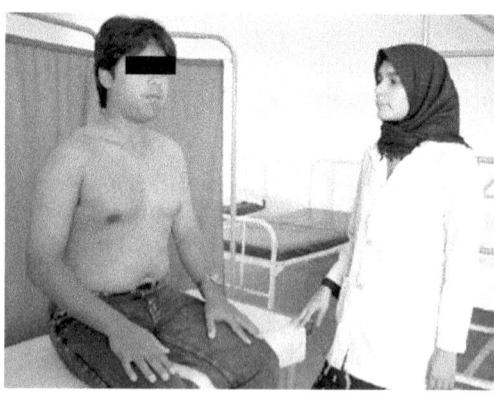

Fig. 9.19: Pursed lip breathing.

procedure is repeated many times with frequent relaxation periods in between.

POSTURAL DRAINAGE

Definition

The postural drainage is the technique of loosening of secretions from the specific areas of the lobes of the lungs.

Anatomy

These are a pair of lungs—the right lung and left lung. The lungs are in turn divided into lobes. The right lung has three lobes—upper lobe, middle lobe and lower lobe. The left lung has two lobes—upper lobe and lower lobe.

Right Lung Lobes

- The upper lobe has three bronchopulmonary segments.
- The middle lobe has two bronchopulmonary segments.
- The lower lobe has five bronchopulmonary segments.

Lobes	Segments
Upper lobe	• Apical • Posterior • Anterior
Middle lobe	• Lateral • Medial
Lower lobe	• Apical • Medial basal • Anterior basal • Lateral basal • Posterior basal

Left Lung Lobes

- The upper lobe has three bronchopulmonary segments.
- The lower lobe has two bronchopulmonary segments.

Lobes	Segments
Upper lobe	• Apical • Posterior • Anterior • Superior • Inferior
Lower lobe	• Apical • Anterior basal • Lateral basal • Posterior basal

Diagnosis

The diagnosis for the requirement of the postural drainage is done by using the radiograph or bronchogram that shows the quantity of the secretions in the lobes.

Indications

1. Chronic diseases: Bronchiectasis, cystic fibrosis
2. Temporary infections: Pneumonia
3. Severe flu or cold to remove excess mucus and clear the lungs.

Contraindications

1. Postural drainage should not be done immediately after the meal as it may lead to nausea and vomiting.
2. Postural drainage should not be performed on the bare skin.

Effects and Uses

The postural drainage uses gravity as the patient is in gravity-assisted position to move the mucus from the lungs to the throat.

Guidelines

1. The patient should be comfortable.
2. The patient should remove the tight clothing, jewelry, buttons around the neck, chest, and waist.
3. The patient should participate actively in the postural drainage.
4. The patient should wear light and soft clothing.
5. The towel is used to decrease the effect of the percussion.
6. The treatment is carried out for a period of about 15-20 minutes.
7. The length of treatment time for each lobe depends upon the amount of secretions present.
8. The lobe which has more secretions should be treated first.
9. The best recommended time for the postural drainage is either early morning or bedtime session.
10. The preparation of the therapist includes removal of jewelries such as rings, watches, and bracelets and maintains the flat and short nails.

Technique

The postural drainage will be more effective if combined with manipulations such as percussion, vibration, deep breathing, and coughing. The total duration for postural drainage is divided equally for each manipulation. It is performed as follows. Each manipulation is performed for 3 to 5 minutes. For example—percussion manipulations like clapping for 3 to 5 minutes, vibration for 15 seconds or vibration for five exhalations followed by coughing or huffing. So all these helps to bring the mucus secretions out of the lungs and cleared. Thus the lungs are cleared or free of secretions.

The patient is positioned on a tilt table and the techniques are started in a sequence at a particular point according to the lobes.

Manipulations

Clapping

The clapping is given on the chest wall over the lung segment to drain the secretions into proximal airway. The clapping is rhythmic and one only over the ribs. Clapping is contraindicated over the spine, stomach and lower ribs, breast bone to prevent injury to the spleen on the left side, liver on the right side, and kidneys on the lower back.

Vibrations

The vibration manipulation is done with the flat hand or by placing hand firmly on the chest wall over the required segment and the therapist tenses his or her muscles of arm and shoulder to create shaking motion followed by this. The therapist applies light pressure over the area that is vibration manipulation is done. Another way of vibration is therapist puts one hand over the other hand and presses the top and bottom hands on each other to vibrate.

Deep Breathing

The patient is suggested to perform the diaphragmatic breathing that helps to loosen the mucus and stimulate coughing.

Coughing

The patient is asked to take deep inspiration followed by expiration with cough. This is important in clearing the airways. The mucus is coughed out. The coughing strain can be reduced to the patient by assisting the supporting the sides of the lower chest with the hands or elbows. This also increases the cough effectiveness.

Huffing

After each position is drained, ask the patient to take deep breath and expire it quickly in a huff. The huff forces the air and the mucus. The huff makes the cough effective.

Duration of the Treatment

The duration is 20-40 minutes.

Position of the Patient

The patient lies on the tilting table. The patient head shoulder be well supported and comfortable position and should also be able to flex his hips and knees for the stronger cough.

Position of the Therapist

The physiotherapist should stand straight, i.e., not in flexed position for longer duration of time or it may lead to low backache.

Equipment Required

1. Drainage tubes
2. Electrical and nonelectrical palm percussions
3. Vibrator

Procedure

The postural drainage is done in the gravity-assisted position. The manipulations such as percussion, vibration are done on the front, back, and side of the patient chest followed by the deep breathing and coughing.

The following is the description of lobes and segments

1. Upper lobe: Apical segment
2. Upper lobe: Posterior segment
3. Upper lobe: Anterior segment
4. Lingula: This is the part of upper lobe of the left lung and has superior and inferior segments
5. Middle lobes of the right lung: Medial and lateral segments
6. Lower lobes: Anterior basal
7. Lower lobes: Posterior basal
8. Lower lobes: Lateral basal
9. Lower lobes: Anterior basal
10. Lower lobes: Posterior basal

Upper Lobe: Apical Segment

Position of the patient
The patient is sitting on the chair with the pillow supporting the back and leaning backward on a pillow at an angle of 30° and should keep both the patient hands on his or her thighs.

Position of the patient
The physical therapist should stand behind the patient.

Technique
The placement of the hand is in between the collar bone and top of the shoulder on both the left and right side of the chest and percussion and vibration are done.

Upper Lobe: Posterior Segment

Position of the patient
The patient sits on a flat table and leans forward on a folded pillow at a 30° **(Fig. 9.20)**.

Position of the therapist
The therapist stands behind the patient.

Technique
The placement of the hand is on the upper back on the left side and right side and the percussion and vibrations are given.

Upper Lobe: Anterior Segment

Position of the patient
The patient is in supine lying on the treatment table with two pillows—one under the head and the other below the hips and knees.

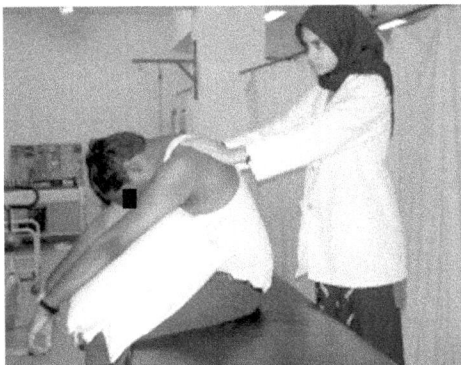

Fig. 9.20: Posterior segment.

Position of the therapist
The physical therapist stands in front of the patient.

Technique
The placement of hands is between the collar bone and the nipple on the both right side and left side of the chest. The percussion and vibrations are done.

Lingula

This is the part of upper lobe of the left lung and has superior and inferior segments.

Position of the patient
The patient is in side-lying with one pillow under the head **(Fig. 9.21)**. The foot end of the table is elevated by 14 in. or 15°. The patient lies on the right side and slightly rotates backwards. This is the proper position for lingual segment of the upper lobes to drain the secretions. A pillow is placed behind the patient from shoulder to the hip and the patient flexes his or her knees.

Position of the therapist
The physiotherapist will be standing behind the patient.

Technique
The hand placement for the men are outside the nipple area on the left side and in women the heel of the hand is placed under the arm pit and fingers are extended below the breast so manipulations are not performed directly on the breast as it would be painful **(Fig. 9.22)**. The percussion and vibration manipulations are done.

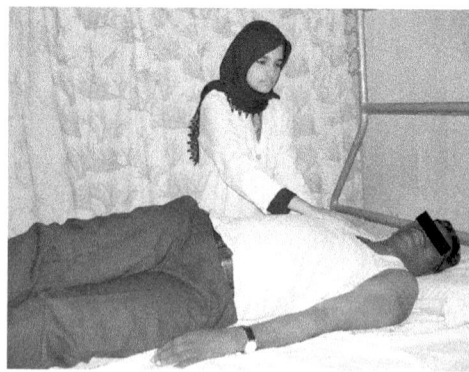

Fig. 9.21: Lingula—position of the patient.

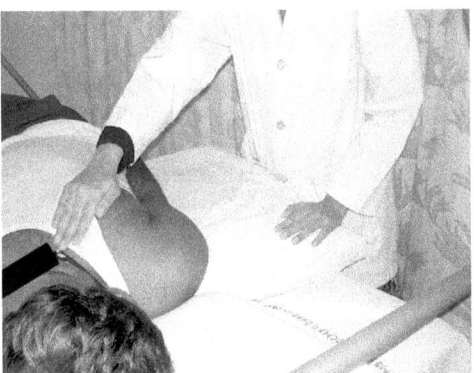

Fig. 9.22: Placement of the hand.

Middle Lobes of the Right Lung

The middle lobe of the right lung consists of medial and lateral segments **(Fig. 9.23)**.

Position of the patient
The tilting table is elevated by 14 in. or 15°. The patient is in side lying with two pillows—one below the head and the other behind the back from shoulder to hip. The patient is asked to flex the knees. The patient lies on the right side and rotates one-fourth backwards towards the left side. This is the proper position for middle lobes of right lung to drain the secretions.

Position of the physical therapist
The physical therapist stands in front of the patient.

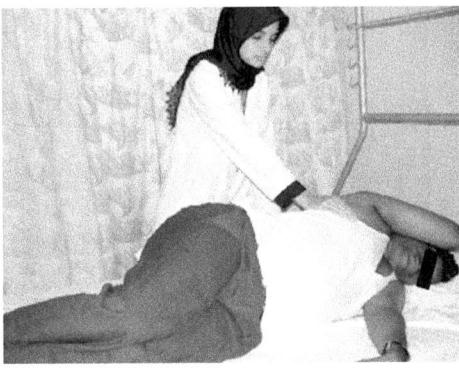

Fig. 9.23: Middle lobe.

Technique
The hand placement for the women are heel of the hand under the armpit and fingers are extended forward beneath the breast. The manipulations are performed and secretions are drained.

Lower Lobes: Left Lung Lower Lobe Anterior Basal Segment

Position of the patient
The treatment table should be elevated by 18 in. or 30°. The patient is in side lying on the right side with one pillow under the head and the other behind the back.

Position of the physiotherapist
The physical therapist stands behind the patient.

Technique
Placement of the hands is on the left side of the lower ribs and percussion and vibration manipulations are given.

Lower Lobes: Posterior Basal: For the Right Lung

Position of the patient
The table is elevated 30° or foot end is raised by 18 in **(Fig. 9.24)**. The patient is in prone lying with two pillows, one below the head and the other below the hips. The patient lies on the abdomen.

Position of the physical therapist
The physical therapist stands beside the patient on the right side.

Technique
The hand placement for the lower lobes of the posterior basal segment of the right lung are on the right side of the patient spine

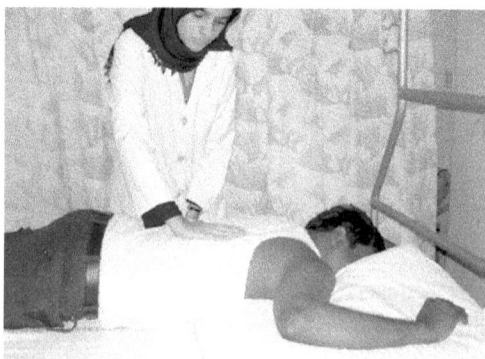

Fig. 9.24: Posterior basal segment.

and the manipulations like percussion and vibration are performed to drain the secretions. Care must be taken not to manipulate spine and lower ribs.

Lower Lobes: Right Lateral Basal Segment

Position of the patient
The treatment table is elevated by 18 in. or about 30° **(Fig. 9.25)**. The patient is in the side-lying position on the left side with two pillows—one under the head and the other in between the flexed knees.

Position of the physical therapist
The physical therapist is standing behind the patient.

Technique
The placement of the hands is on the uppermost portion of the lower ribs. The percussion and vibration manipulations are given over the uppermost portion of the lower right ribs.

Lower Lobes: Right Lung Lower Lobe Anterior Basal Segment

Position of the patient
The treatment table should be elevated by 18 in. or 30°. The patient is in side lying on the left side with one pillow under the head and the other behind the back.

Position of the physical therapist
The physical therapist stands behind the patient.

Technique
Placement of the hands is on the right side of the lower ribs and percussion and vibration manipulations are given.

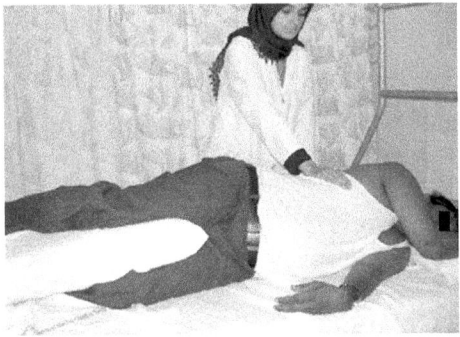

Fig. 9.25: Right lateral basal segment.

Lower Lobes: Posterior Basal Segment for the Left Lung

Position of the patient
The table is elevated 30° or foot end is raised by 18 in. The patient is in prone lying with two pillows, one below the head and the other below the hips. The patient lies on the abdomen.

Position of the physical therapist
The physical therapist stands beside the patient on the left side.

Technique
The placement of the hands on the left side of the patient's spine and the percussion and vibration manipulations are done. Care must be taken not to manipulate spine and lower ribs.

Lower Lobes: Left Lateral Basal Segment

Position of the patient
The treatment table is elevated by 18 in. or about 30° **(Fig. 9.26)**. The patient is in the side-lying position on the right side with two pillows, one under the head and the other in between the flexed knees.

Position of the physical therapist
The physical therapist is standing behind the patient.

Technique
The placement of the hands is on the uppermost portion of the lower ribs. The percussion and vibration manipulations are given over the uppermost portion of the lower left ribs.

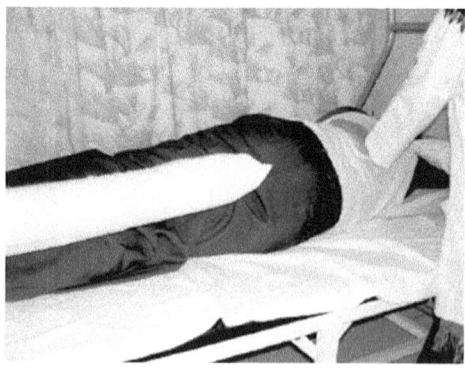

Fig. 9.26: Left lateral basal segment.

Lower Lobes: Right Apical Segment

Position of the patient
The patient is in the prone lying on the abdomen on the flat table with two pillows under the hips.

Position of the physical therapist
Standing beside the patient on the right side in walk standing position.

Technique
The placement of the hands is over the middle part of the back at the bottom of the shoulder blade on the right side. Extra care is to be taken the manipulations are not performed on the spine.

Lower Lobes: Left Apical Segment

Position of the patient
The patient is in the prone lying on the abdomen on the flat table with two pillows under the hips.

Position of the physical therapist
Standing beside the patient on the left side in walk standing position.

Technique
The placement of the hands is over the middle part of the back at the bottom of the shoulder blade on the left side. Care to be taken that manipulations are not done on the spine.

THORACIC EXPANSION EXERCISE

Aim

1. To mobilize secretions
2. To improve ventilation
3. To prevent atelectasis
4. To re-expand collapsed alveoli

Technique

The patient is in comfortable position (**Fig. 9.27**). The patient is asked to breathe in slowly and deeply through the nose and breathe out through the mouth. The patient is asked to inspire the maximum air, ask the patient to inspire for the second time. The physical therapist places the hands on the chest wall where the expansion occurs and a quick stretch to inspiratory muscles is applied. The therapist quickly squeezes the patient chest wall between the therapist hands at the

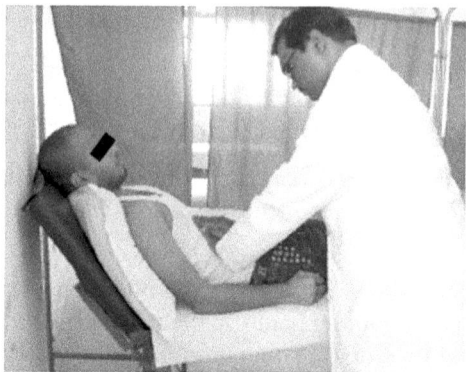

Fig. 9.27: Half lying thoracic expansion exercise.

beginning of the inspiration and releases the pressure and patient is asked to inspire maximum air possible.

This is explained to the patient and physical therapist should give maximum resistance to the maximum volume. The resistance initially should be stronger and later should decrease.

This inspired air improves ventilation to the peripheral areas by mobilizing the mucus plugs and secretions.

The thoracic expansion exercises are combined with postural drainage, chest shaking, and vibrations or with the active cycle of breathing technique. This can be done unilaterally or bilaterally. This combination is very effective for the patient.

INHALATION THERAPY

The inhalation therapy is used to break up the mucus and to induce the relaxation in bronchial smooth muscle by using the bronchodilators.

This is done by:
1. Aerosol
2. Nebulizer

These both can be given during intermittent positive pressure breathing or steam inhalation.

Aerosol

Aerosol is the commonly used handheld device. The patient should be trained with the proper use of the aerosol so patient inhales the maximum amount of medication into the lungs and avoid the loss of the drug into atmosphere. Usually 10% of the drug reaches the bronchi and 90% of the drug is swallowed. To ensure maximum amount of the drug reaches the bronchi, the drug should be released at the beginning of the inspiration.

The patient should take a gap of 1 minute before starting with the next inspiration. Few patients will be on both bronchodilators and steroid therapy using aerosols. Then, the bronchodilators should be administered first so that airways get dilated. Give a gap of 15–20 minutes then steroid therapy can be started depending upon the type of the drug used.

Rotahaler

The patient should be well trained how to handle the Rotahaler properly. Initially, the capsule should be inserted. The capsule has colored end. It is an indication that end has to be inserted first in to Rotahaler and Rotahaler is twisted so the capsule is broken and patient is asked to inhale deeply to get the medication into the major airways for effectiveness. The patient is asked to breathe several times to inhale the drug completely.

Other Types of Inhaling Devices

Spinhalers

This is the device advised for the children and the use is similar to the Rotahaler.

Spacer

The spacer is a different type of device used for the patients who cannot inspire medication. So in the spacer there is a mouthpiece and the mouthpiece is depressed. So the patient will be able to inhale the drug.

Nebuhaler

The nebuhaler is an aerosol where the mouthpiece helps to deliver the drug. When the patient is willing to take medication the nebuhaler is depressed into the patient's mouth so the drug is released.

Nebulizer

This is another device for inhalation therapy where the drug is broken into the fine particles to enhance the inhalation. It is administered by compressed oxygen or air. The patient's position should be relaxed and comfortable with well supported by the pillows. The patient has a choice of using either face mask for the young patients or disabled breathless patients and mouthpiece for the patients who can hold the mouthpiece with the lips to deliver the drug. The patient when inhales the drug by inhaler. The medication will take 10 to 15 minutes for completely reaching the lungs so the patient is asked to perform relax breathing followed by 1 or 2 deep breaths so the drug presentation occurs completely into the airways.

Types of Nebulizer

1. In one type of nebulizer, the steam of gas is passed through a hole that creates a low pressure. This is passed through the tube where the other end is immersed in bronchodilator solution. The liquid passes through the tube and gets split into the small pieces and nebulizer is ready for use.
2. **Nebulizer with piezoelectric effect:** The liquid is moved by a vibrating crystal. This type of nebulizer is used for home purpose. This delivers high humidity for patients with thick sputum to aid expectoration.

HUMIDIFICATION

Principle

The air is moistened because it is passed through water vapor. The patient is asked to inspire the air by face mask or by the mouthpiece. Normally, the air passing through the nose and pharynx is continuously moistening the respiratory mucous. If this is inefficient, the cilial action is impaired and secretions are viscid so there is a need of humidification to loosen the viscid and thick secretions.

Humidification is the moistening of the air and gases, this is the normal function of the upper respiratory tract; if this is inefficient, then artificial humidification is required.

Indications

1. When the patient is breathing through the tracheostomy tubes or endotracheal tubes. The patient feels the dry air that has a temperature less than the body temperature. The secretions in the bronchial tree takes the moisture and form crusts. The crusts block the trachea and it in turn blocks small airways, the ciliary action and humidification is lost so patient requires artificial humidification.
2. Artificial humidification is required for the patient who are using the oxygen masks. The oxygen masks consist of the dry air so

leads to lack of humidification. So artificial humidification is required.
3. Artificial humidification also helps in excretion of thick secretions.

Choice of Humidifiers

1. The patient with dry gases used ultrasonic type of humidifier.
2. The patients need disposal humidified which can deliver < 28% of oxygen. This type of humidifier is indicated for patients with respiratory failure secondary to chronic bronchitis, asthma and emphysema.

Methods

a. The humidification is given by the wide boring tube.
b. A short period of humidification is given before the chest clearance is done for the patient who is not intubated but breath freely. This is nebulizer method with a face mask and mouthpiece.
c. For the patient with tracheostomy tube or endotracheal tube, a Brompton tube (a tracheostomy humidifying tube T tube) is used. This is a plastic tube and can fit into humidification wide boring tube. Other one is disposable tracheostomy mask made of plastic which is flexible.
d. A patient with intermittent positive pressure ventilation also needs humidification. For this patient, humidifiers are fitted with the ventilators. So heated humidifiers of about 34 + or −2°C are used and kept at the endotracheal tube or tracheostomy.

Types

The humidifiers are called suppliers and are divided into four types. They are:
1. Ambient temperature vapor suppliers
2. Heated vapor suppliers
3. Ambient aerosol suppliers
4. Heated aerosol suppliers

1. **Ambient temperature vapor suppliers:** In this type, the humidification is obtained through the water with tiny gas bubbles at room temperature
2. **Heated vapor suppliers:** In this type, the hot water is taken with gas and patient's tube is heated in Fisher-Paykell device to prevent temperature loss. A thermometer is attached so it gives feedback about the delivering the gas at over 39°. The

thermometer has cuff-off mechanism. If temperature is more than 39° the patient will not be able to tolerate and cuff off mechanism of the thermometer will get disconnected and gas is delivered back once the temperature reaches 39°.
3. **Ambient aerosol suppliers:** This works on the Bernoulli principle. The subtypes of the aerosols are Bird, ohio, bard inspiron. The mist of the liquid water is produced in three ways:
    i. High-pressure gas jet on an anvil
    ii. High-speed spinning disc
    iii. Ultrasonic vibratory crystal

    The recent ambient aerosol suppliers work on the Babington principle. The air is forced through a fine film of water that produces dense mist and gas is delivered to the patient.
4. **Heated aerosol suppliers:** In this type, the heated water is used along with nebulizing drug. This also works on Bernoulli principle and care of thermal safety is taken and patient is delivered gas.

INTERMITTENT POSITIVE PRESSURE BREATHING

This is also called intermittent positive pressure ventilation. This is the assisted inspiration. The air under pressure by pressure cycled ventilators such as Bird and Bennett enters the bronchial tree and mobilizes the secretions and increases the aeration of the alveoli. The patient with bronchospasm can use the bronchodilator drugs. The ventilators are set in such a way that the assisted inspiration with intermittent positive pressure ventilation occurs along with patient's normal breathing pattern.

To Remove the Secretions

Effective Coughing

Definition
The coughing is the forced expiration technique against a closed glottis.

Aim
To clear the secretions from the trachea and bronchi.

Technique
The patient is asked to take deep breath, then tighten the abdominal muscle, and cough. The air is breathed is high lung volume and deep breath.

Effects and uses: The coughing clears the secretions from the central airways.

Huffing

Definition
This is the forced expiration with the glottis open.

Aim
To move the secretions from the smaller bronchi to larger bronchi.

Technique: The patient is asked to breathe in and tighten the abdominal muscle and huff through the mouth. The air is breathed in mid lung volume to breathe is medium sized.

Effect and uses
The secretions are moved from the peripheral airway.

Forced Expiratory Technique

Aim
1. To mobilize the secretions from the peripheral airways to the proximal airways **(Fig. 9.28)**.
2. To decrease bronchospasm.

Technique
The patient is asked to perform 1 or 2 huffs, relaxed breathing, and once or twice coughing.

The huffing is done from the mid lung volume to the low lung volume so that the secretions are moved from the peripheral airway.

The coughing is performed at the high lung volume and clears the secretions for the central airway.

The relaxed breathing is to decrease or prevent the bronchospasm.

The patient is asked to take a medium size of air to breathe in followed by a forced expiration through the mouth open. Then the patient is asked to huff once or twice and then breathing control.

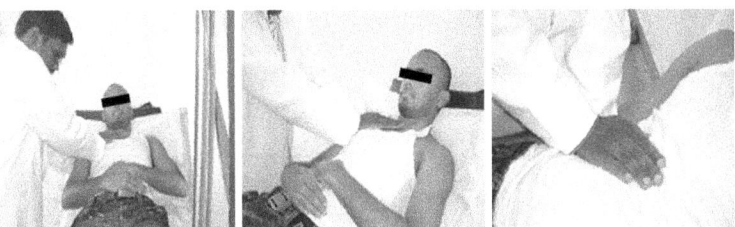

Fig. 9.28: Forced expiratory technique.

The technique must be repeated till the secretions are reached the proximal airways then followed by a cough of high intensity to remove secretions. This technique can also be combined with the active cycle of breathing technique to be most effective.

Active Cycle Breathing Technique

Aim
To clear bronchial secretions.

Position of the patient
Less secretions: Sitting.

More secretions: Alternate side lying combined with postural drainage

Total treatment time
It is 15–30 minutes.

Technique
The active cycle breathing technique is combined with the thoracic expansion exercise, breathing control, forced expiratory technique with huffing or coughing.

The patient is asked to perform the controlled breathing then three or four thoracic expansion exercises then forced expiratory technique. The techniques are performed initially with mid-to-low lung volume and once the secretions have reached the proximal airway then coughing or huffing with high lung volume is done to remove the bronchial secretions.

Self-treatment regime
The patient is trained and encouraged to perform the technique on his own so that the patient can practice in the time of emergency and as a home program too **(Fig. 9.29)**.

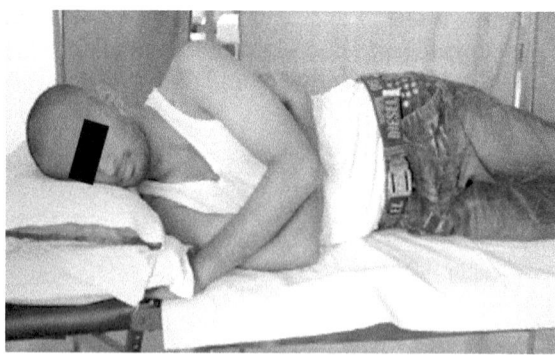

Fig. 9.29: Side-lying patient is practicing the self-treatment regime.

Suction

Aim
To remove the accumulated secretions from the main bronchi, tracheas and pharynx.

Technique
A catheter is passed through the pharynx or nasopharynx or can be done through endotracheal tube or tracheostomy tube.

This catheter on the other end is attached to the suction pump and the secretions are sucked out. The suction is done by respiratory therapist.

Postural Drainage

The patient can practice lying on a bundle of newspapers and the attendant can perform the percussion manipulation and the patient can perform coughing and huffing.

Breathing Exercise

The patient can perform all types of breathing exercises and resistance can be offered by using the webbing belt.

Loosening of the Secretion

The patient can perform thoracic expansion exercises.

Sputum Disposal

This is done by techniques such as coughing, huffing, and forced expiratory technique.

Regular exercise regime can be planned.

Postural awareness in all activities of the daily living.

Cardiopulmonary Resuscitation 10

◼ DEFINITION

Cardiopulmonary resuscitation (CPR) is the emergency lifesaving technique performed on the patient when the heart stops to beat. When there is a cardiac arrest the immediate cardiopulmonary resuscitation is done so the chances of the survival is high. CPR is the technique for re-establishing heart and lung action after cardiac arrest or apparent sudden death resulting from electric shock, drowning, respiratory arrest, and other causes.

Recognize cardiac arrest, activate emergency response system: early CPR with chest compressions, rapid defibrillation, emergency medical services both basic and advanced, advanced life support, and post-cardiac arrest care.

The cardiopulmonary resuscitation is done by the trained personnel only. It includes chest compression, mouth to mouth breathing at the rate of 30:2 compression to breaths. The chest compressions are 100 to 120 beats/min and depth of 2 inches. When there is sudden cardiac arrest is seen at home, work and park, first emergency call has to be made then while emergency personnel are on their way then hands only CPR is performed until they arrive.

Cardiopulmonary resuscitation is of three types:
1. Basic life support (ABC)
2. Advanced life support (DEF)
3. Prolonged life support (GHI)

Basic Life Support (ABC)

A: Airway: Airway ensures that patient has patent airway. Remove fluid and debris from the mouth if present.

B: Breathing: Breathing is the maintenance of a patent airway. Inflation of patient's lungs is done rapidly 3.5 times using the following methods:
1. Use mouth-to-mouth or nose-to-mouth ventilation.
2. An airway is inserted to provide mouth to airway ventilation.
3. Ventilate the patient using a bag and mask.

C: Circulation: Control bleeding by applying pressure on bleeding point and elevate it.

Advanced Life Support (DEF)

D: Drugs:
- Adrenalin—0.5-1 mg, repeated 3-5 minutes
- Sodium bicarbonate 1 mEq/kg body weight, repeated every 10 minutes of arrest time
- Intravenous fluid as required, e.g., blood or plasma

E: ECG: ECG must be monitored as soon as possible.

F: Fibrillation treatment:
- External defibrillation using 100-400 J. Repeat shock as necessary.
- Convert fine fibrillation to coarse fibrillation using adrenalin.
- Administer lignocaine 1-2 mg/kg intravenously as necessary.

Prolonged Life Support (GHI)

G: Gauging:
- Gauge the likely outcome of resuscitation.
- Gauge the cause of the cardiorespiratory arrest and treat it.

H: Human mentation:
- Preserve cerebral suction by maintaining normal cerebral blood flow and oxygenation.
- Reduce and control intracranial pressure.
- Monitor cerebral function.

I: Intensive care:
- Provide intensive therapy
- Intensive nursing
- Intensive monitoring

COMPONENTS OF CARDIOPULMONARY RESUSCITATION

The two major components of the CPR are described in the following sections:

Cardiac Massage

Indications

- Cardiac arrest causes cessation of heartbeat that will lead to cerebral anoxia and patient dies within 3 minutes.
- Circulatory arrest and disappearance of the carotid pulse indicates cerebral anoxia.

Procedure: Airway must be clear so that oxygen reaches the lungs. The surgeon begins external or internal cardiac massage.

External Cardiac Massage

In this the heart is compressed between the sternum anteriorly and vertebral column posteriorly. The pericardium restricts lateral movement. The natural elasticity of the thoracic cage permits 4 to 5 cm depression or the sternum before any damage is done to the ribs or the costal cartilages. As the compression is released, the natural elasticity of heart sucks blood from the great veins and blood flow is seen in the ventricles.

The patient is placed supine on a firm surface. The surgeon places the heel of one hand over the lower part of the sternum but superior to xiphisternal joint. The other hand is placed on the top of this hand and pressure is applied vertically downward on the sternum approximately every second. After each pressure, the surgeon allows the chest to re-expand fully. Sixty compressions are attempted in 1 minute.

In small children, only one hand is used and sternum is depressed with the thumb. After immediate threat to the life is removed, ECG is done and cardiac monitor is attached. In ventricular fibrillation, electrical defibrillator should be carried out.

Internal Cardiac Massage

When there is no reaction of the heart to the massage then the external cardiac massage is failed then the internal cardiac massage is planned. This is done by thoracic or abdominal approach. There is another option of using Transabdominal route and this is preferred only when positive pressure ventilation and endotracheal intubation are absent.

Transthoracic approach: The patient left arm is abducted and surgeon stands on the left side of the patient. An incision is made at the left fourth intercostal space. The pleura is opened, heart is protected. The right hand of the surgeon is insinuated into the thoracic cavity and by placing the palm beneath the heart it is compressed against the sternum at the rate of about once a second.

This is continued till the surgeon gets pain in his hands when the hands are withdrawn and the costal cartilages are divided above and below. A mechanical rib retractor is used to retract the ribs apart.

Cardiopulmonary Resuscitation

Pericardium is opened as quickly as possible in front of left phrenic nerve. The cardiac massage is restarted with the right hand behind the heart and left hand in front of it. The compression should be gradual and relaxation abrupt. The heart must be full before it can be emptied again. The compression should be made evenly with the palmar surfaces of the fingers and care must be taken not to injure the heart by using the tip of the fingers.

If the heart is blue and flaccid and for continuing systole 5–10 mL of 1% calcium chloride is injected directly into the left ventricle. For continuing the systole the heart should be pink and heart should have tone. If there is no heart tone then 1–2 mL of 1:1000 adrenalin is injected into the left ventricle. As this solution induce fibrillation patient may need electrical defibrillator. Patient is given sodium bicarbonate intravenously and the dosage is 100 to 150 mL. Followed by this the pericardium is repaired, internal mammary arteries are ligated, suturing is done around the ribs and chest drainage is connected to the water seal drainage.

Subdiaphragmatic Cardiac Massage

A midline upper abdominal incision is made. The hand is introduced and compression is carried out through the diaphragm. The massage can be improved if the diaphragm is opened. The triangular ligament of the left lobe of liver is divided. The diaphragm and pericardium are incised to expose the heart. The opening is enlarged. The fingers are insinuated through this opening, and with palmar surface of fingers, the heart is compressed against the sternum. The required time is 80 minutes of cardiac massage.

Defibrillation

Automated external defibrillator (AED): This increases the survival rate of the victim. It guides how to use AED program. This is performed by trained personnel only. When ventricular fibrillation occurs, ECG will show irregular low-amplitude wave line at the place of regular QRS complex. Once this is recognized, electrical defibrillation should be attempted. One electrode is applied to the anterior chest wall to the right side of the sternum other over the cardiac apex. Direct current of 200 J is used and shock is given or alternate current of 300–750 V is used. After a brief period of a systole, the heart will revert to the normal rhythm. If heart fails to revert, higher voltages are required. A further period of massage may convert fine fibrillation into coarse one. A volume of 5 mL of calcium chloride (10%) given directly to the heart will improve myocardial tone. Normal contraction of the heart persistently reverts to ventricular fibrillation, and then procaine amide or lignocaine (1 mL/kg body weight) should be injected.

The heart should be observed for a sufficiently longer time period of about 20 minutes.

Artificial Ventilation/Respiration

Artificial respiration is a lifesaving measure.

Indications

- Acute asphyxia due to drowning
- Gas poisoning
- Electrocution
- Anesthetic accidents

Method

Mouth-to-mouth breathing.

Advantages

Simple method, works by expanding the lungs.

Procedure

The victim should be in supine position the airway should be opened by placing a hand under the neck and lifting. Keeping pressure on forehead with the other hand, extend the neck and lift the tongue away from the back of the throat. The victim's mouth is covered by the operator's mouth. The operator blows about 12 times a minute into the victim's mouth. The tidal volume becomes twice. Elastic recoil of lungs causes passive expiration. The victim's neck is kept extended. For apnea patients both artificial respiration and cardiac massage are performed together.

Mechanical Respirators

Indications

- Chronic respiratory insufficiency
- Pulmonary edema
- Acute respiratory distress syndrome

The mechanoreceptors are airtight metal or plastic containers that are used to enclose the body except head. Portable covers only the chest. The mechanical respirators has motor that creates negative pressure that is applied to the chest at regular intervals so the movement can be brought into the chest wall. When the patient breaths against positive end expiratory pressure prevents respiratory distress syndrome.

Complications
- Weak and malnourished patients.
- When respirometer takes over the work of breathing, there is disuse atrophy of the respiratory muscles.

Relaxation Techniques   11

■ DEFINITION

The ability to relax is called relaxation. It is the technique where the mind and body are free from anxiety and tension. Relaxation occurs in the frontal lobe of the brain. Relaxation helps in reducing stress, anxiety, anger, and fear. Relaxation is spending quiet times, listening to music, or reading a book, and be away from other distractions of one's life. Relaxing the body and mind creates a sense of well-being. It allows physical recovery and helps to prevent the tension. When the mind is relaxed the body is also relaxed, so body and mind are closely linked. Stress and worry can manifest as headache or backache, while physical pain or exhaustion increases worry and stress. Everyone should try to find a little time everyday to relax themselves. By doing this, everyone will feel more energetic for their work. When the patient gets adequate sleep. The sleep relaxes the body.

Steps for Relaxation

There are four basic steps to practice relaxation. They are quiet and peaceful environment, comfortable position, instrumental music, and positive stress.

Practicing Relaxation

Relaxation is very simple. The art of relaxation lies in taking time for practicing. Relaxation can be practiced for a period of 15–20 minutes in the morning, or after returning from work, or after bath, or before going to the bed. Relaxation time is always useful .Relaxation relieves the person from stress and helps to cope up with all the activities of daily living.

Types of Relaxation

There are three types of relaxation. They are:
1. Mental Relaxation
2. Physical relaxation
3. Progressive muscle relaxation.

Mental Technique

This relaxation technique is basically meditation. It decreases psychological and physical stress, e.g., hypnosis gives deep state of relaxation. This is helpful to reduce pain, to lessen smoking addiction, for patients undergoing chemotherapy treatment, to lose weight, to relieve allergy and rash, to decrease body metabolism, to manage blood pressure, to relieve muscle tension, to control heart rate and pulse, to calm breathing activity, and to increase immune response. Mental health is important for day-to-day activities. It also decreases stress and helps overcome negative thoughts.

Physical Technique

This techniques includes breathing exercises and progressive muscle relaxation techniques. The first technique is practicing breathing exercises that decreases stress. Deep abdominal breathing decreases anger, anxiety, depression, and hypertension. The second technique is progressive muscle technique that focuses on muscles from top to bottom: flexing, holding, and relaxing the muscle. It improves physiological, mental, and physical health, best example is it reduces insomnia. Physical health is important for daily work. It also reduces blood pressure, respiratory rate, heart rate, and metabolism.

Progressive muscle relaxation technique

The individual is supine lying or half lying, and the mind is concentrated on normal breathing. All the major and minor parts are mentally viewed; their shapes are recalled and visualized, i.e., visualize each part of the body and relax each part of the body while visualizing and follow the sequence.

Upper limb
Begins with thumb-fore finger-middle finger-ring finger-little finger-back of the palm-the palm-wrist-forearm-upper arm-shoulder (both sides).

Lower limb
Begins with big toe-second toe-third toe-fourth toe-little toe-the upper part of the foot-sole-heel-ankle-calf-knee-thigh-thigh joint (both sides).

Back
From the bottom of the backbone to the neck-the right side of the back-the back of the right shoulder-the left side of the back-the back of the left shoulder-the back of the neck.

Abdomen chest and throat
Begins from navel-the left side of the navel (including urinary organs)-the right side of the navel-the upper side of the navel-the central part of the chest-right breast-left breast-the pit below in the throat.

Head
Begins from chin-lower lip-tongue-right nostril-right cheek-right ear-right eye-left eye-left ear-left cheek-left nostril-tip of the nose-the center of the eyebrows-forehead-right side of the head-back of the head-left side of the head-top of the head.

Each part should be concentrated for 10-20 seconds. The shape should be visualized by mind with closed eyes. While doing so, the concentration spot should be completely relaxed. The entire process should be completed in about 15-30 minutes, this will complete one round.

Therapeutic/Physiological Relaxation

This is basically used by health-care professionals, such as counselors and psychologist. They also prescribe the medication if required. This technique is nervous system relaxation. This relaxation increases resistance power of immune system. Example: Cancer and AIDS patients (acquired immunodeficiency syndrome).

Other Relaxation Techniques

The relaxation can be practiced anywhere, any time in positions such as sitting and supine lying positions. They are:
1. Raise your shoulders up toward your ears, count 5, and go back to initial position.
2. Bring shoulders to front and then back to normal. Repeat it for five times.
3. Try to bring both the eyebrows near to each other as if you are frowning, press your lips and tighten your eyes, hold them and count 5, and then release them.
4. Relax all the features of the face one by one.

Breathing techniques and general relaxation are very much useful for the individual. The breathing technique is one of the stress free and relaxation induced techniques. Take time in a day and try to spend minimum of 10 minutes or more on focused relaxation. Find a quiet spot and lie comfortably with a small pillow under head, lose your idea and try to imagine each part of your body and relax them part by part.

Advantages of Relaxation

1. It helps in relieving stress and tension.
2. It helps in getting peaceful sound sleep.
3. Mind and body gets complete rest.
4. Quality of sleep improves, sleep duration is reduced, and time is saved.
5. Tiredness of the body is relieved.
6. All the parts of the body are relaxed to their maximum and are recharged with energy.
7. Tension, anxiety, depression, stress, strain, negative thoughts, and high blood pressure are controlled.
8. The individual feels physically stable and mentally peaceful.
9. Memory, willpower, inner energies, and knowledge are developed.
10. Regular practice and focus helps to improve concentration, meditation and self realization.

Breathing Control Techniques — 12

▮ INTRODUCTION

The breathing control techniques are helpful for the patients who are suffering from breathlessness. The inspiratory muscles like diaphragm fill the lungs with air and release it gradually. Exercises for breathing control improve lung capacity. Respiratory control center is located at the base of the brain in medulla and pons. The main function of the respiratory center is to control the breathing, e.g., breathing rate such as holding your breath or faster breathing.

Aims

1. To reduce bronchospasm
2. To improve the reduced work of breathing
3. To encourage the slow respiratory rate
4. To encourage increased tidal volume

Indications

1. Wheeze
2. Severe breathlessness

Duration

The duration depends on how the patient feels and the duration of breathlessness. Active cycle of breathing techniques are one of the types of breathing control techniques. Usually, the patient is asked to perform 6 breaths.

Patient Instructions

Patient is asked to breathe in and out by nose; if it is not possible, the patient is asked to breathe out by mouth using pursed lip breathing.

The patient is also asked to release the tension of their body with each breathing. The shoulders should be relaxed, making breathing slowly.

If possible the patient is asked to close his/her eyes to focus on breathing and then relax. Breathing control techniques continues until the patient feels relaxed.

Contraindications

Unconsciousness, unable to follow the instructions, confused, or agitated patient.

Various Positions to Practice Breathing Control

The following are the alternate positions the patient should be taught to practice breathing control:
1. Relaxed half-lying
2. Supported forward leaning
3. High side lying
4. Relaxed sitting
5. Forward lean standing
6. Back lean standing
7. Side lean standing

Relaxed Half-lying

The patient is in half-lying position and relaxed. The physical therapist places one hand on the patient's upper abdomen just below the xiphisternum to check the rise and fall of the patient's breathing pattern and the patient is taught the technique of the breathing pattern.

Supported Forward Leaning

The patient sits on a chair and leans forward on the table with four pillows **(Fig. 12.1)**. The three pillows are placed on the table, then patient is asked to keep both the upper extremities on top of three pillows and the fourth is placed on the top of upper extremities and patient is asked to lie on the fourth pillow.

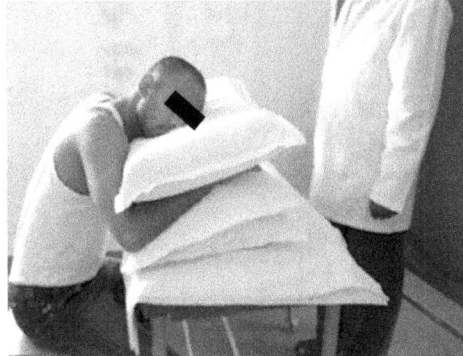

Fig. 12.1: Supported forward leaning position.

High Side Lying

The patient is in side-lying position, e.g., if the patient is lying on the right side, the left upper extremity is placed as follows: shoulder adducted, internally rotated, elbow slightly flexed, forearm pronated, and wrist and fingers are slightly flexed and placed on the anterior aspect of the chest **(Fig. 12.2)**. Three pillows are required; two are placed under head and the third on the couch below the right upper extremity. The placement of the right upper extremity is as follows: shoulder is abducted to 90°, externally rotated, elbow flexed, forearm supinated, and wrist and fingers extended.

Relaxed Sitting

The patient sits on the stool and slightly bends the spine forward **(Fig. 12.3)**. The patient is relaxed. The head is bent forward, both the

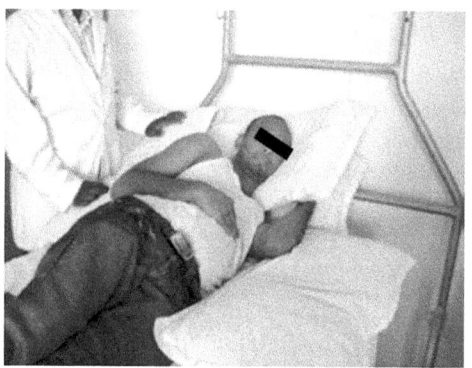

Fig. 12.2: High side-lying position.

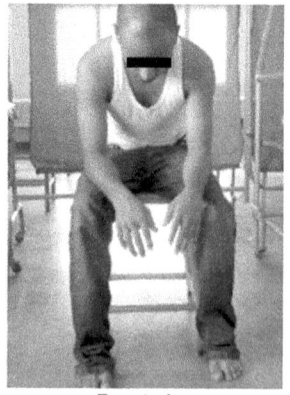 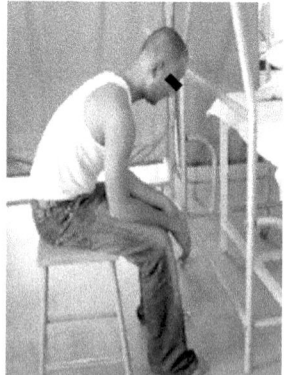

Front view   Side view

Fig. 12.3: Relaxed sitting.

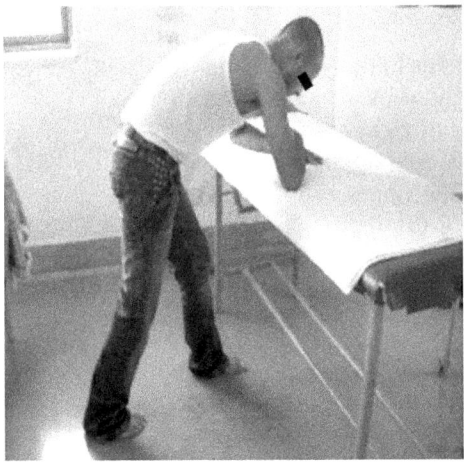

Fig. 12.4: Forward lean standing position.

upper limbs are relaxed on the thighs, shoulders are flexed, elbows are slightly flexed, forearm are pronated, and wrist and fingers are flexed.

Forward Lean Standing

The patient is in the walk-standing position in front of the couch, trunk, shoulders and elbows are flexed, forearms are supinated, and wrist and fingers are slightly flexed **(Fig. 12.4)**. The forearm, wrist, and fingers are relaxed on the couch and the wrists of the both hands are crossed.

Back Lean Standing

The patient is in standing position with legs placed wide **(Fig. 12.5)**. The patient's back touches the wall from behind and trunk is slightly flexed. The upper extremities are placed as follows. The shoulders are adducted, internally rotated, elbows are slightly flexed, forearm in mid-prone position, wrist are extended and fingers are flexed and placed on the thighs.

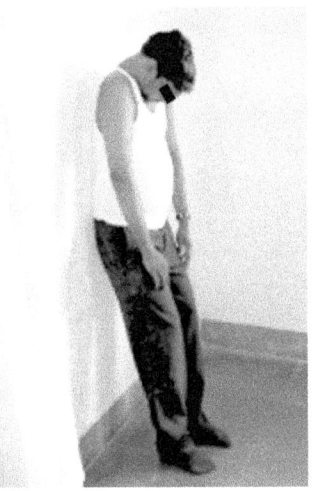

Fig. 12.5: Back lean standing.

Side Lean Standing

The patient leans to the wall on one side either right or left, e.g., while the patient leans to right side, his/her head is flexed, right upper extremity is extended, left upper extremity is slightly flexed, the right side lower extremity the knee is flexed and left side lower extremity where the knee is extended **(Fig. 12.6)**.

Uses of Breathing Control

- Improves lung ventilation
- Clear and loosen the secretions from the lungs
- Improve cough effectiveness
- Airway relaxation
- Relieve tightness after coughing or breathlessness
- Relieve wheezing; shortness of breath, anxiety, and fear.

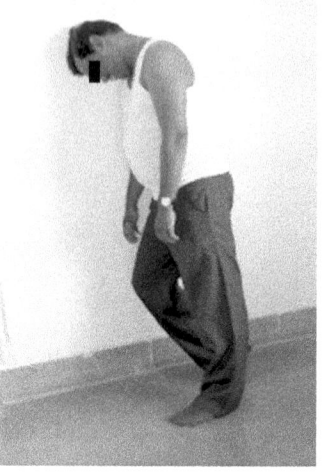

Fig. 12.6: Side lean standing.

Posture

CHAPTER 13

DEFINITION

The position where body is held.

TYPES

Static Posture

Holding the body when not moving, e.g., sleeping, sitting, and standing.

Dynamic Posture

Holding the body when moving, e.g., picking up object and bending forward, running, and walking.

Good Posture

Always keep chest, back, shoulder forward with head upright and spine in line.

Bad Posture

Hunching forward and slouching forward. The bad posture causes joint and muscle pain.

FACTORS AFFECTING

Posture is affected with decreased muscle strength, scoliosis, improper sitting, standing and head forward, sitting at the desk for long time and looking at the smart phone, tiring/extra work out, unbalanced training.

EXERCISES TO CORRECT POSTURE

Reverse Plank Bridge

This helps in strengthening of muscles such as middle trapezius, rhomboids, erector spine, and neck flexors and stretching the muscles such as pectoralis, biceps, deltoid, and neck extensors, and during this technique, bring back hands and fingers. This posture emphases two more muscles. They are external rotators and biceps.

Arch Up

This is posterior tilting of the pelvis. The muscles strengthened are shoulder flexors, horizontal abduction like rhomboids and middle trapezius, shoulder extensors such as deltoid, neck flexors. Muscles stretched are neck extensors, internal rotators, and thoracic spine extensors such as erector spinae.

Rows

Rows are performed using dumbbells and barbells. This is by bringing shoulder blades together and shoulder in backward position.

MUSCLES AFFECTING POSTURE

Core stability muscles or postural muscles are the deep muscles of the back, pelvis, abdomen. The muscles are multifidus, transverse abdominis, pelvic floor, gluteus and hamstrings. To maintain the erect posture the following exercises help and the following muscles work. The exercises and muscles are:
1. Single leg extension to stabilize the pelvis.
2. Crunch exercises work on rectus abdominis and oblique muscles.
3. Pilates roll up or yoga sit ups works on rectus abdominis, oblique and transverse abdominis.
4. Cross over works on obliques.
5. Back extension for erector spinae.
6. Plank pose for obliques, transverse abdominis, shoulder muscles and back muscles.

POSTURAL DEFORMITIES

Kyphosis

Hunching of the back, it is excess outward curvature of the spine. Treatment is strengthening abdominals and back muscles.

Lordosis

It is excess inward curvature of the spine. Causes are weak hamstrings and tight hip flexors. Treatment is for strengthening hamstrings and stretching hip flexors.

Scoliosis

It is sideward curvature of the spine.

Causes are muscular dystrophy and cerebral palsy. It occurs before puberty due to growth spurt so kids should be screened for scoliosis. Treatment can be done before the progression of the condition.

Scheuermann Disease

This is front to back curvature of the spine which occurs due to spondylolisthesis.

Flat Foot or Pes Planus or Fallen Arches

This is the postural deformity where foot arches are collapsed so entire sole of the foot is in contact with the ground.

Causes for this condition are diabetes, obesity, pregnancy, aging, muscular dystrophy, and cerebral palsy.

Treatment is done using pain medications such as NSAID, physical therapy treatment includes RICE (Rest, Ice application, Compression, and Elevation) to reduce pain and swelling, orthotic devices, shoe modification, if the inflammation continues then corticosteroids injections are given to reduce the inflammation. Once the pain and inflammation is reduced, then exercises such as heel stretches, tennis/golf ball rolls, arch lifts, calf raise, stair arches raise, towel curls, and toe raises are to be performed. Each exercise is performed for 2-3 sets for 10-15 repetitions.

Knock Knees/Genu Valgum

The knees are together and feet and ankles are apart. This increases pain on the front of the knee. Causes are rickets (Vitamin D and calcium deficiency) treatment is surgery. Physical therapy also helps in correcting the condition during initial stages such as exercises to strengthen the hip, thigh and leg muscles, stretching the tight adductors. Few exercises are done using barbells rotating on inner thigh and using massage tools for trigger points. Stretching adductors in sitting with forearm pushing on thighs, butterfly stretch, prone adductor stretch and side splits. All stretches are for 30-60 seconds and for 4-5 sets.

Bow Legs /Genu Varum

The knees are outward and ankle and foot touch each other.

Commonly seen in infants and toddlers but requires treatment if the same continues for 4 years.

In adult the cause is osteoarthritis. If severe deformity occurs, osteotomy is the treatment but if deformity is because of the posture, the following exercises can help. When the hip adductors are weak, these muscles should be strengthened using Theraband, weights of about 2 lb to 5 lb depending on the capacity of the person. Usually start with less weight and gradually increase the weight or muscles will get fatigued the hip abductors and external rotators are tight so stretch these two group of muscles. The self-stretching is performed and stretch is hold for 5 to 10 seconds, followed by this relax and perform stretch again.

Total Body Exercises, Muscles and their Functions

14

INTRODUCTION

A full-body exercise is working on a variety of muscle groups such as head and neck, upper body, lower body, and core muscles. All the exercises help in increasing the aerobic activity and strengthening the various groups of muscles in the whole body. They also help to maintain the vital signs like heart rate, oxygen saturation, blood pressure and respiratory rate. The ideal duration of the exercise depends on the individual, age, medical diagnosis. Recommended aerobic activity for an average person should be at least 30 to 60 minutes per day considering all the criteria. Muscle-strengthening exercises uses various sets and repetitions. A set is a certain number of repetitions; a repetition is the total motion of an exercise with frequent rest periods. All exercises should start with less number of sets and repetitions which gradually should increase. If a person does intense exercise, it can lead to muscle ache for the first time then a rest day is given for the muscles to recover. Hence, slow and gradual increase in the intensity of exercise is advisable so as to prevent injury.

NECK EXERCISES

Neck Flexion

Neck Flexors

There are superficial and deep neck flexors.

The superficial neck muscles are sternocleidomastoid. They are located on either side of the neck. They basically has two major functions. They are in bilateral neck flexion and ipsilateral lateral flexion and contralateral neck rotation and anterior scalene.

Deep neck flexors are the longus colli, longus capitis, longus cervicus, and rectus capitis. These four muscles helps in maintaining good neck posture and stability.

Procedure

Maintain the neck in neutral position, breathe out and bend your head forward so as the chin touches the chest. Hold it for five seconds and take a deep breath and bring back the neck to the initial position.

Neck Extension

Neck Extensors

The muscles are levator scapulae, upper trapezius, splenius cervicis, splenius capitis, semispinalis cervicis, and semispinalis capitis.

Procedure

Maintain the neck in neutral position, breath out, extend the neck and breathe in, and bring the neck into the starting position.

Neck Lateral Flexion or Side Bending

Lateral Flexors

Sternocleidomastoid helps for ipsilateral lateral flexion and contralateral rotation.

Procedure

Maintain the neck in neutral position, breath out, bend the neck to the right side and breathe in, and bring the neck into the starting position. Repeat the same on the left side.

Neck Rotation

Neck Rotators

The action of the neck muscles are sternocleidomastoid helps in rotating the neck to the contralateral or opposite side. The splenius muscles perform multiple actions like extending the neck or backward bending the neck, lateral flexion of the neck or side bending the neck and rotating the neck or turning the neck to the same side.

Procedure

Maintain the neck in neutral position and then rotate the neck or turn the neck to the right side and then bring the neck back to the starting position or midline and perform the same on the left side. Followed by this perform total circles of the neck in clockwise direction and anti-clockwise direction. Each direction rotation is performed for three times.

▍SHOULDER GIRDLE EXERCISES

The shoulder girdle consists of five joints. They are glenohumeral joint (shoulder joint), scapulothoracic joint, acromioclavicular joint, sternoclavicular joint, and coracoacromial arch. The bones are mainly scapula and humerus attached to sternum and clavicle.

Scapula, Muscles and Movement

There are four movements: elevation, depression, protraction, and retraction.

Sitting

The patient should be relaxed; straighten the spine, head should be straight, and both hands on the thighs. The following exercises are to be practiced.

Elevation of the shoulder girdles
Raise both the shoulder girdles toward the ear lobe. Make sure the neck and trunk are also straight.

Muscles: Levator scapulae, trapezius, rhomboids major and minor.

Depression of the shoulder girdles
Lower both the shoulder girdles away from ear lobes muscles: Towards the direction of force of gravity.

Muscles: The muscles helping are pectoralis major and minor, serratus anterior, and latissimus dorsi.

Protraction of the shoulder girdles
Bring both the shoulder girdles forward towards the sternum.

Muscles: Pectoralis major and minor and serratus anterior.

Retraction of the shoulder girdles
Bring the shoulder girdles back towards the scapula.

Muscles: Latissimus dorsi, trapezius, and rhomboids major and minor.

Standing

The patient should be standing with feet separated and practice the following exercises.

Elevation of the shoulder girdles
Raise both the shoulder girdles toward the ear lobe.

Depression of the shoulder girdles
Lower both the shoulder girdles away from the ear lobe.

Protraction of the shoulder girdles
Bring both the shoulder girdles in front towards the sternum.

Retraction of the shoulder girdles
Bring the shoulder girdles back towards the scapula.

SHOULDER EXERCISES

The functions of the shoulder are flexion, extension, abduction, adduction, internal rotation, and external rotation.

The exercises can be performed in both short lever and long lever and in all the positions mentioned below.

Supine Lying

The shoulder and elbow should be straight or elbow should be extended and the whole upper extremity should move as a single unit.

Long-lever Exercises

Flexion of the Shoulder

Shoulder is moved forward and raised up to 180°.

Muscles
Anterior deltoid, coracobrachialis, and pectoralis major.

Abduction of the Shoulder

Shoulder is taken away from the body up to 180°.

Muscles
Supraspinatus (0–15°), deltoid (15–90°), trapezius, and serratus anterior (90–180°).

Adduction of the Shoulder

Shoulder is moved towards and across the body.

Muscles
Latissimus dorsi, teres major, teres minor, subscapularis, long head of triceps, infraspinatus, and coracobrachialis.

Side Lying: The Top Shoulder Should be Moved

Flexion of the Shoulder

Shoulder moved in front up to 180°.

Extension of the Shoulder

Shoulder is moved back until 70–80°.

Muscles

Latissimus dorsi, teres major, teres minor, and posterior deltoid.

Abduction of the Shoulder

Shoulder is moved away from the body up to 180°.

Adduction of the Shoulder

Shoulder should be moved toward and across the body.

Short-lever Exercises

Sitting

The patient will be sitting on the stool. The patient elbow is flexed and fingers should touch the shoulder.

1. **Flexion of the shoulder:** Raise both the upper extremities.
2. **Extension of the shoulder:** Take the upper extremities backward.
3. **Abduction of the shoulder:** Move the upper extremities away from the body.
4. **Adduction of the shoulder:** Move the upper extremities towards the body.
5. **Rotation of the shoulder:** Circle the upper extremities in the clockwise direction.
6. **Rotation of the shoulder:** Circle the upper extremities in the anticlockwise direction.

Standing

1. **Flexion of the shoulder:** Raise both the upper extremities.
2. **Extension of the shoulder:** Take the upper extremities backward.
3. **Abduction of the shoulder:** Move the upper extremities away from the body.
4. **Adduction of the shoulder:** Move the upper extremities toward the body.
5. **Rotation of the shoulder:** Circle the upper extremities in the clockwise direction.
6. **Rotation of the shoulder:** Circle the upper extremities in the anticlockwise direction.
7. **Internal rotation:** Turning the shoulder internally or inward. *Muscles:* Subscapularis.
8. **External rotation:** Turning the shoulder externally or outward.
9. **Muscles:** Teres minor and infraspinatus.

10. **Rotator cuff:** The four muscles form rotator cuff. They are supraspinatus, infraspinatus, subscapularis, and teres minor. All the above muscles help to depress the humeral head against the glenoid cavity by keeping the shoulder joint intact.

Elbow Exercises

- **Elbow flexion:** Bend the elbow toward the shoulder.
  Muscles: Biceps brachii, brachialis, brachioradialis.
- **Elbow extension:** Straighten the elbow to initial position.
  Muscles: Triceps, anconeus.
- **Supination:** Turn the forearm with the palm facing upward direction.
  Muscles: Supinator, biceps brachii.
- **Pronation:** Turn the forearm with the palm facing downward direction.
  Muscles: Pronator teres, pronator quadratus.

Wrist Exercises

- **Wrist flexion:** Bend the wrist towards the palm.
  Muscles: Flexor carpi radialis, flexor carpi ulnaris, flexor digitorum superficialis.
- **Wrist extension:** Bend the wrist away from the palm.
  Muscles: Extensor carpi radialis longus, extensor carpi radialis brevis, extensor carpi ulnaris, extensor digitorum.
- **Radial deviation:** From the midprone position rotate the palm facing downward.
  Muscles: Flexor carpi radialis, extensor carpi radialis longus and extensor carpi radialis brevis.
- **Ulnar deviation:** From the midprone position rotate the palm facing upward.
  Muscles: Flexor carpi ulnaris, extensor carpi ulnaris.

Finger Exercises

- **Finger flexion:** Bend the fingers toward the palm.
  Muscles: Flexor digitorum superficialis, flexor digitorum profundus.
- **Finger extension:** Bend the fingers away from the palm.
  Muscles: Extensor digitorum.
- **Finger abduction:** Move the fingers away from the middle finger.
  Muscles: Dorsal interossei.
- **Finger adduction:** Move the fingers toward the middle finger.
  Muscles: Palmar interossei.

Trunk Exercises

Standing
The patient should be standing with a wide base and hands are placed on the waist.
1. **Trunk flexion:** Breathe out and bend forward, breathe in and come to the starting position.
   Muscles: External and internal obliques, rectus **abdominis**, erector spinae, semispinalis thoracis, latissimus dorsi, quadratus lumborum, and psoas major.
2. **Trunk extension:** Breathe out and bend backward, breathe in and come to the starting position.
   Muscles: Erector spinae or sacrospinalis, quadratus lumborum.
3. **Trunk lateral bending to the right side:** Breathe out and bend to the right side, breathe in and come to the starting position.
   Muscles: Erector spinae, internal and external oblique, quadratus lumborum.
4. **Trunk lateral bending to the left side:** Breathe out and bend to the left side, breathe in and come to the starting position.
   Muscles: Erector spinae, internal and external oblique, quadratus lumborum.

Sitting
The patient is sitting on the stool with feet wide apart.
1. **Trunk flexion:** Breathe out and bend forward, breathe in and come to the starting position.
2. **Trunk extension:** Breathe out and bend backward, breathe in and come to the starting position.
3. **Trunk lateral bending to the right side:** Breathe out and bend to the right side, breathe in and come to the starting position.
4. **Trunk lateral bending to the left side:** Breathe out and bend to the left side, breathe in and come to the starting position.
5. Sitting with fists on the side of the chest wall and trunk bending sideways.

Pelvic Girdle

The patient is in crook lying (supine lying with hips and knees flexed). Whenever the movement is performed, raise the pelvis up from the couch.
1. Move the pelvis forward.
2. Move the pelvis backward.
3. Move the pelvis right side.
4. Move the pelvis left side.

Pelvic bridging exercise

The patient is in crook lying. The physiotherapist should stabilize the knee and the feet. The patient is asked to raise the pelvis above the couch and count 10. Repeat the same for 3–4 repetitions, relax, and perform 3–4 sets.

Muscles: The following muscles are stretched. They are gluteus medius, gluteus maximus, and hamstring and stabilizing muscles are quadriceps, rectus abdominis, and oblique muscles.

Standing: The patient will be standing with a wide base with both the hands on the pelvis and perform pelvic rotation, both clockwise and anticlockwise directions.

Lower Limb

Supine lying

The patient is in supine lying with both the lower extremities straight or extended.

1. **Hip flexion:** Raise the lower extremity toward the ceiling.
   Muscles: Iliacus and psoas major.
2. **Hip abduction:** Take the lower extremity away from the midline.
   Muscles: Gluteus medius, gluteus minimus, and tensor fascia lata.
3. **Hip adduction:** Bring the lower extremity toward the midline.
   Muscles: Adductor longus, adductor brevis, and adductor magnus.

Side lying

The patient is in side lying with both lower extremities extended or straight. The lower extremity on the top should be exercised.

1. **Hip flexion:** Move the lower extremity forward.
2. **Hip extension:** Move the lower extremity backward. Muscles: Hamstrings.
3. **Hip abduction:** Raise the lower extremity away from the midline.
4. **Hip adduction:** Raise the lower extremity toward the midline.

Knee Exercises

Supine lying

The patient is in supine lying with both the lower extremities straight or extended.

1. **Knee rolling side to side**
2. **Flexion of the knee:** Bend the knee. Muscles: Hamstrings
3. **Extension of the knee:** Straighten the knee. Muscles: Quadriceps

Perform the same on both the side separately.

Sitting

The patient will be in a high sitting position:
1. **Flexion of the knee:** Bend the knee.
2. **Extension of the knee:** Straighten the knee.

Ankle and Foot

Supine lying
1. **Dorsiflexion:** Bend the foot forward.
   Muscles: Tibialis anterior, extensor halluces longus, extensor digitorum longus, peroneus tertius.
2. **Plantar flexion:** Bend the foot backward.
   Muscles: Tibialis posterior, flexor hallucis longus, flexor digitorum longus, gastrocnemius, soleus, peroneus.
3. Foot circling in forward and backward direction.

All the exercises should be performed for about five repetitions each and about 3-5 sets with frequent relaxation periods. The repetitions and number of sets should be increased gradually. Warm-up and cooldown stretching exercises should be performed before and after the exercise program.

Home Management

The home exercise program is designed with a series of exercise for the patient to perform at home to maintain the strength, endurance, and to increase the therapeutic gains. Home exercise program is designed so that the patient can maximize the efforts and continue to get the benefits.

Glossary

Acute: Sudden or severe illness of short duration.
Acute bronchitis: A respiratory tract infection that causes inflammation of the trachea and the bronchi.
Aneurysm: A bulge or swelling in an artery that has been weakened by disease or injury.
Angina pectoris: Angina pectoris pain is felt as dull pressure or pain in the center of the chest that radiates towards the left arm.
Angiocardiography: An X-ray examination of the heart and its blood vessel by injecting a substance.
Angiography: An X-ray examination of blood vessel.
Angioplasty: The surgical technique for repairing of damaged blood vessels.
Aorta: The main artery of the body that extends from the left ventricle of the heart and distributes blood throughout the body.
Arrhythmia: An irregular heartbeat.
Arteriosclerosis: This is a condition where the walls of the arteries are thickened leading to decreased blood supply to the organs and whole body.
Artery: The vessel that deliver blood from the heart to throughout the body.
Atherosclerosis: A condition of the arteries in which blood flow is blocked by fatty deposit.
Auscultation: Listening to sounds of heart and lungs with the aid of the stethoscope.
Blood: Blood is a body fluid which circulates and delivers oxygen and nutrients to the body cells. Blood consist of four components. They are plasma, red blood cells, white blood cells and platelets.
Blood vessels: The arteries, veins, and capillaries that carry blood.
Bronchitis: The inflammation of the bronchi or air passages of the lungs.
Bypass: Bypass grafting is a surgical technique performed for cardiovascular conditions like blockage of arteries where a section of artery is taken and attached around the clogged section of the artery for passage of blood .
Capillary: The extremely tiny blood vessel that connects the arteries and veins.

Glossary

Cardiology: The study of heart and circulating system especially diagnosis and treatment of disorder.
Cardiopulmonary resuscitation: The use of artificial ventilation to revive from the cardiac arrest.
Cardiovascular system: The system that circulates blood to all cells.
Chest: The chest is formed by 12 pairs of ribs attached anteriorly to the sternum and posteriorly to the vertebrae.
Chest cavity: The chest cavity is occupied by heart and lungs.
Circulating system: The circulating system carries blood from organs to all parts of the body.
Congenital: Existing from birth.
Cystic fibrosis: Cystic fibrosis is a lung condition developing during childhood age, which affects the function of the respiratory system and sweat glands causing abnormal production of the mucous.
Decortication: The removal of outer layer of an organ.
Defibrillation technique: This technique is used to correct abnormal heartbeat.
Diaphragm: The muscular partition that separates the chest cavity and the abdominal cavity.
Embolism: The blockage of the blood vessel by an obstruction called embolus.
Emphysema: A lung condition in which the air spaces in the lungs are enlarged
Extrasystole: An abnormal contraction of the heart.
Heart: Heart is a muscular organ helps in the circulation of the blood throughout the body.
Heart attack: A sudden diminishing of the hearts ability to function.
Heart murmur: An abnormal heart sound that can be detected by stethoscope.
Hypertension: High blood pressure.
Hypotension: Low blood pressure.
Ischemia: The tissue death because of loss of blood supply.
Myocarditis: The inflammation of the myocardium.
Pacemaker: An artificial device that stimulates heart action and regularizes the heart beat by the periodic discharge of electrical impulses.
Respiration: Inhalation and exhalation of air is called respiration.
Respiratory arrest: A cessation of breathing.
Respiratory system: Respiratory system consists of nose, throat, larynx, trachea, bronchi and lungs. The main function of the respiratory system is exchange of the gases.

Shock: Shock is the life threatening situation caused due to insufficient blood flow through the body occurs secondary to severe illness or injury.

Sneeze: An involuntary action that causes sudden force of air through noise and mouth for expelling irritants.

Sphygmomanometer: A device for measuring blood pressure.

Tachycardia: Abnormal rapid heartbeat.

Thoracotomy: It is the surgical opening of the chest or thorax for performing correction surgery of the lungs.

Thrombosis: Coagulation of the blood.

Thrombus: A blood clot formed in the heart or blood vessel.

Trachea: The tube that extends from the larynx to the bronchi in the respiratory tract.

Vein: The vessel that carry blood back to the heart.

Wheeze: Difficulty in breathing that is accompanied by a whistling sound.

Index

Page numbers followed by *f* refer to figure.

A

Abdominal symptoms 115
Acquired immunodeficiency syndrome 310
ACSM
 leg ergometer equation 245
 stepping equation 247
 walking equation 244
Acute respiratory distress syndrome 306
Adequate airway, maintenance of 192
Adequate gas exchange 167
Adrenalin 303
Adson test 144
Aerobic capacity 252
Aerosol suppliers
 ambient 298
 heated 298
Air, density of 40
Airflow resistance 38
Airway clearance techniques 36, 225
Airway resistance 38, 40
 factors affecting 40
Allen maneuver 145
Alveolar ventilation 43
Ambient temperature vapor suppliers 297
Amplitude 73
Anesthetic accidents 306
Aneurysm 330
Angina 232
 nocturnal 116
 pectoris 116, 232, 330
 postinfarction 117
 prinzmetal 117
 stable 116
 unstable 117
Angiocardiography 330
Angiography 152, 330
Angioplasty 232, 330

Ankle
 and foot 329
 circles 201
Anomalies of cervical rib, types of 8
Anxiety 309
Aorta 330
 coarctation of 84
 injury, ascending 138
 over-riding of 99
 rupture of 137
Aortic arch injury 141
Aortic opening 8
Aortic regurgitation 91, 111
Aortic rupture, ascending 141
Aortography 138
Apical breathing
 left unilateral 275*f*
 right unilateral 275*f*
Arrhythmia 65, 92, 232, 330
 cardiac 72
 ectopic 66
 normotropic 66
 types of 66
Arterial stiffness 31
Arterial supply 3, 25
Arteriosclerosis 330
Arteriovenous malformation 103
Artery 330
Aspergillosis 171
Asphyxia, acute 306
Asthma 53, 218, 223
 atopic 223
 attack 41
 cardiac 115
 extrinsic 223
 intrinsic 224
 nonatopic 224
Astrand-Rhyming step test protocol 249
Atherosclerosis 77, 330

Index

Atrial extrasystole 67
Atrial fibrillation 68, 78, 105
Atrial flutter 68
Atrial septal defect 91
Atrioventricular malformation 91
Atrioventricular node 26
    paroxysmal tachycardia 68
Auscultation 198, 330
Autogenic drainage 228
Automated external defibrillator 305
Avoid low calorie diet 49

B

Babington principle 298
Back 309
    lean standing 315, 315f, 316f
    strengthening exercises 161
Backache 308
Balloon
    angioplasty 232
    valvuloplasty 80, 107
Baroreceptors 32
Basal metabolism 47
Basal segment
    left lateral 292f
    right lateral 291f
Bench stepping submaximal test 249
Bilobectomy 177
Bipolar leads 75
Bleeding site, identifying 166
Blood 166, 330
    circulating in blood vessel, amount of 31
    gases, altered 115
    supply 1
    test 210
    vessels 173, 330
Blood pressure 30, 81, 91, 110, 238, 239
    control of 32
    decreased 114
    diastolic 32
    factors affecting 31
    systemic arterial 32
    systolic 32
Blunt injury 132
Body, tissues of 49
Bone
    deformity 12
    pain 12

Bony cage 8
Bony thorax and lungs 4
Bow legs 319
Brachytherapy 175
Bradycardia 65, 239
Brain, higher centers of 33
Breathing 22, 38
    bilateral
        apical 275, 276f
        costal 276, 277f
        posterior basal 279, 279f
    control 299, 312
        and techniques 312
        phase 36
        practice 313
        uses of 316
    diaphragmatic 273, 273f, 274f
    disorders of 38
    exercises 221, 223, 225, 271, 309
    factors affecting 38
    force 23
    glossopharyngeal 281
    lingular 280, 280f
    mouth-to-mouth 306
    muscles, overloading of 23
    pattern 55
    pursed lip 282, 282f
    quiet 22
    rate 55
    segmental 274
    self-apical 275f
    self-costal 278
    self-pursed lip 282
    shortness of 92
    sounds 55
    techniques, active cycle of 36, 300, 312
    types of 22
Breathlessness, duration of 312
Bronchial injury 148
Bronchial muscle, tone of 40
Bronchial tree 2
    functions of 3
Bronchiectasis 167, 218, 226, 229
    sicca, causes for 163
Bronchitis
    acute 330
    chronic 53, 218, 219
Bronchography 166, 227
Bronchopleural fistula 154

Index

Bronchopneumonia 170
Bronchopulmonary segments 3
Bronchoscopy 166, 174
Bronchostenosis 164
Bronchus, injury to 137
Bundle branch block 67
Bundle of His 26
Bypass grafting 330

C

Calcium chloride 306
Capillary 330
Cardiac arrest 180, 302
Cardiac catheterization 95, 98, 101, 108
Cardiac dysrhythmia 181
Cardiac failure 92, 117
   acute 117
   chronic 117
   congestive 117, 181
Cardiac massage 303
   external 304
   internal 304
   subdiaphragmatic 305
Cardiac output 31
Cardiac rehabilitation 120, 231
   exercise program 212, 233
   inpatient 213, 233
Cardiac rehabilitation program 119, 121, 231
   categories of 232
   indications of 232
   phases of 121
Cardiac rhythm, disorders of 115
Cardiac surgery 77, 91
Cardiac tamponade 150, 181
Cardiology 331
Cardiopulmonary resuscitation 302, 331
   components of 303
Cardiorespiratory fitness 252
   test 239
Cardiovascular function 167
Cardiovascular system 331
Carotid sinus syncope 71
Carpal tunnel syndrome 10
Central chemoreceptors 29
Cerebral anemia 81, 110
Cerebral symptoms 115
Cerebral syncope 71

Cervical rib 8
   with local symptoms 9
   with nerve pressure symptoms 9
   with vascular symptoms 9
Chemoreceptors 28, 29, 33
Chemotherapeutic agents 175
Chemotherapy 168, 175
   postoperative 175
Chest 4, 310, 331
   cavity 331
   flail 124
   funnel 8, 14
   infections 92
   leads, unipolar 76
   mobility 223
   pain in 114
   percussion 221
   physical therapy 35, 126
   shape 54
   stove in 126
   trauma 132
   wall 39
      mobility exercises 221
      oscillation, high frequency 38
   X-ray 56, 79, 81, 103, 106, 110, 174
Chronic obstructive airway disease 218
Chronic obstructive pulmonary disease 218, 256
   assessment for 61
   types of 62
Circulatory complications 187
Circus movement 68
Clamminess and sweating 114
Clapping 268, 268f, 285
Clubbing 54
Coarctation, types of 85
Color Doppler 84
Combination therapy 175
Computed tomography 174
Computerized spirometer 60, 263
Concurrent chemoradiotherapy 176
Congenital conditions 91
Conservative physical therapy 87, 120
Conservative treatment 211
Contusion 150
Coronary angiogram 119
Coronary artery
   bypass surgery 66, 232

disease 91, 113
injury 151
Coronary sinus defects 91
Costoclavicular syndrome 145
Coughing 201, 285
    effective 298
    reflex 34
    syncope 71
    techniques 221
Curative treatment 101
Cyanosis 54, 100
Cystic fibrosis 218, 228, 331
    physical therapy treatment for 230

D

Decortication 156, 331
Deep breathing 22, 201, 285
    benefits of 22
Deep vein thrombosis 140, 186
Defibrillation 305
    technique 331
Defibrillator 212
Deformity 14, 19
Dependent program techniques 35
Depression 309
Diabetes mellitus 232
Diagnostic peritoneal lavage 151
Diaphragm 8, 331
    large openings in 8
Diaphragmatic fatigue 23
Diffusion 41
    abnormalities 43
    values of 41
Digestive complications 188
Digital subtraction angiograph 86
Disability 265
Discontinuous tests 242
Distal innominate artery 141
Distance run tests 250
Dock's sign 85
Doppler study 98
Doppler's effect 108, 113
Dorsiflexion 329
Douglas bag 48
Droopy shoulder symptoms 145
Drowning 302
Dynamic compliance 39
Dyspnea 92, 100, 114

E

Echocardiogram 79, 82, 84, 92, 95, 98, 101, 103, 106, 108, 111, 112, 118
    with Doppler 95
Echocardiography 210
    and color Doppler 86
    and Doppler effect 118
Ectopic beat 68
Ectopy
    supraventricular 68
    ventricular 69
Edema 54, 114
Effort syncope 71
Elasticity 38
Elbow
    exercises 326
    extension 326
    flexed 314
    flexion 326
Electrical conduction abnormality, physical therapy treatment for 69
Electrocardiogram 27, 151
    changes 210
Electrocardiograph 27, 71
    leads 75
Electrographic grid 73
Embolism 106, 111, 331
Emotion 48
Emotional syncope 70
Emphysema 41, 218, 221, 331
Empyema 2, 152, 182
    acute 153
    chronic 156
    latent 154
    persistent 154
    sub-acute 154
    types of 153, 154
Endocrine abnormalities 173
Endomyocardial fibrosis 77
Endonasal tube 202, 204, 205
    complications of 205
Endotracheal intubation 304
Endotracheal tube 202, 205
    complications of 205
    description of 204
    functions of 203
Endurance training 23
Energy conservation 223

Index

physical therapy management
for 47
techniques for 257
Energy expenditure 46, 47
Energy metabolism, determination of 48
Esophageal opening 8
Eupnea 22
Exercise 20
   abnormal 239
   aerobic 221
   cardiac response to 238
   full-body 321
   knee 328
   long-lever 324
   muscle-strengthening 321
   prescription 252
   program 18
   short-lever 325
   spinal stabilization 161
   thoracic expansion 37, 293
   to correct posture 317
   to increase energy expenditure 49
   tolerance 56
   total body 321
Exercise test 61, 264
   bench stepping maximal 246
   bicycle ergometer maximal 245
   bicycle ergometer submaximal 249
   guidelines of 242
   maximal 241, 243
   protocol 241
   submaximal 247, 250
   treadmill submaximal 247
Exertion 100
Expiration
   deep 21
   phase of 40
   quiet 21, 22
Expiratory muscle 22
   training 23
Expiratory reserve volume 57
External rotators 320
Extrasystole 331
Extubation 207
   steps for 208
Exudative stage 152

F

Fallen arches 319
Fallot's spells 100
Fatigue 12, 92
Fibrillation 65
   treatment 303
Fibrinolytic therapy 133
Fibrinopurulent stage 152
Field test 250
   additional 251
Finger
   abduction 326
   adduction 326
   exercises 326
   extension 326
   flexion 326
Fisher-Paykell device 297
Fissures 2
Flat foot 319
Flow resistance 23
Fluids and electrolyte 193
Flutter 65
Food, energy values of 46
Forced expiratory
   flow 58
      rate 261
   technique 37, 299, 299f
Forced vital capacity 259
Forearm supinated 314
Forward lean standing position 315f
Fossa ovalis defect 91
Functional residual capacity 57, 60, 263, 264

G

Gas transfer tests 61, 264
Gastric distention 193
Gauging 303
Genu
   valgum 319
   varum 319
Gradual occlusion 115
Great vessels
   dextro-transposition of 102
   injury to 137
   levo-transposition of 102
   transposition of 91, 102

Index

H

Haemophilus influenzae 227
Half-lying thoracic expansion exercise 294*f*
Hand 54
  placement of 289*f*
Handicap 266
Head 310
Headache 308
Healthy adults, energy expenditure in 46
Heart 24, 331
  and lung action, re-establishing 302
  attack 331
  block 67, 115
    complete 67
    incomplete 67
    third-degree 67
  conditions, closed 77, 87
  conducting system of 26
  disease
    acquired 77
    congenital 77, 232
    ischemic 113
    rheumatic 77, 232
  failure 232
    congestive 232
    right 78, 105
  injury 137, 150
  murmur 92, 331
  nerve supply of 25
  palpitation 92
  rate 238
  rupture 116
  stab injury of 150
  transplant 232
  valves of 24
Heated vapor suppliers 297
Helium dilution technique 60, 263
Hematemesis 54
Hemopneumothorax 134, 150
Hemoptysis 115
  massive 165
  pseudomassive 165
Hemorrhage, pulmonary 166
Hemorrhagic diathesis 166
Hemothorax 2, 132, 150, 182
High frequency positive 194

High side-lying position 314*f*
Hip
  abduction 328
  adduction 328
  flexion 328
  pain 12
Histoplasmosis 164
Huffing 286
Human mentation 303
Humidification, artificial 296
Humidifiers, choice of 297
Hunter syndrome 77
Hydropneumothorax 2
Hyperabduction syndrome 145
Hypercapnia 182
Hyperpnea, voluntary isocapnic 23
Hypertension 33, 331, 232, 309
  pulmonary 78, 91, 105
Hypotension 33, 331
Hypoventilation 43
Hypoxemia 43
Hypoxia 42, 183

I

Illness, acute 232
Incentive respiratory spirometry 281
Incentive spirometry 201
Independent program techniques 35
Induction chemotherapy 176
Infection 134, 229
  pseudomonas 53
Infranodal block 67
Inhalation therapy 294
Inhaling devices 295
  nebuhaler 295
  spacer 295
  spinhalers 295
  types of 295
Inspiration 21
  cycling to 197
  deep 21
  forced 21
  phase of 40
  quiet 21, 22
Inspiratory capacity 57
Inspiratory muscle 22, 312
  training 23, 225
Inspiratory reserve volume 57
Intracoronary imaging 152

Index

Intravenous fluid 303
Intubation, steps of 205
Ischemia 331

J

Joint stiffness 187
Jugular venous pressure 55

K

Knock knees 319
Kyphosis 8, 15, 18, 318
   first-degree 19
   second-degree 19
   third-degree 19

L

Large arteries, elasticity of 31
Larynx 166
Lateral costal breathing 276
   belt exercises for 278*f*
Lateral incisions 178
Left ventricular failure 211
Life support
   advanced 302, 303
   basic 302
   prolonged 302, 303
Lingula 288*f*
Lobectomy 177, 188
Lobes 2
   lower 290-293
   middle 289, 289*f*
   upper 287
      anterior segment 287
      apical segment 287
      posterior segment 287
Lordosis 15, 318
Low compliance 39
Lower limb 309, 328
Lown-Ganong-Levine syndrome 68
Lung 2
   abscess 169
   capacities 57, 261
   carcinoma of 172
   compliance 38
   contusion and laceration 135
   elastic fibers of 39
   injury 150
   lobes
      left 283
      right 283
   suppurative lesions of 167
   tissue, abnormal development of 229
   ventilator, independent 196
   volumes 57
Lutembacher's syndrome 77
Lymphatic drainage 1, 3, 25

M

Magnetic resonance imaging 174
Main pulmonary artery 177
   injury 139, 142
Main stem bronchus 177
Maitland techniques 161
Mandatory ventilator, controlled 195
Manipulations 267, 285
   type of 267
Max-Planck respirometer 48
Mechanical respirators 306
Mechanical ventilator, controlled 195
Medial border 144
Median sternotomy 179
Medical management of rickets 12
Mental relaxation 308
Metabolic calculation 243
Metabolic rate
   basal 49
   basic 48
Micturition syncope 71
Minitracheostomy 206
Mitral regurgitation 91, 107
Mitral stenosis 77, 91, 104
   clinical features of 78
   complications of 78
   diagnosis of 79
   medical treatment for 79
   surgical treatment for 80
   types of 78, 105
Monitoring devices 199
Motor neuron disease 10
Movement, principles of 20
Mucoviscidosis 228
Muscle 323, 324
   affecting posture 318
   contraction, electrical changes during 72
   group of 320, 321

supplying thorax 7
    weakness 12, 187
Myocardial infarction 209, 232
Myocarditis 331
Myocardium 26, 209
    electrical activity of 26

N

Nasal intubation 203
Nasogastric tube complications 205
Nebulizer 294, 295
    types of 296
Neck
    exercises 321
    extension 322
    flexion 321
    flexors 321
    lateral flexion 322
    rotation 322
Needle aspiration biopsy 166
Negative pressure 194
Neoplasm 133
Nerve supply 1, 3
Neurally medicated syncope 71
Neurocardiogenic syncope 71
Nitrogen washout method 60, 264
Nodal extrasystole 67
Non-ST segment myocardial infarction 211
Nontraumatic pneumothorax 129

O

One-mile jogging test 251
Open heart
    conditions, acquired 119
    surgery 232
    surgical conditions 91
Open pneumothorax 128
Open valvotomy 80
Oral airway oscillation devices 37
Oral intubation 203
Osteoarthritis 320
Osteomalacia 8, *11*, 12

P

Palliative radiotherapy 175
Palliative treatment 101
Pallor 54, 81, 110

Palpation 55, 198
Paracentesis thoracis 2
Parasympathetic nerve supply 25
Partial atrioventricular canal defect 91
Patent ductus arteriosus 82
Pectoralis syndrome 145
Pectus carinatum 13
Pelvic
    bridging exercise 328
    girdle 327
Pelvis 318
Penetrating cardiac injury 149
Percussion 55, 198
Percutaneous needle biopsy 174
Perfusion 41, 44, 45, 46
Pericardial rub 114
Pericardial tamponade 150
Pericardium 305
Peripheral chemoreceptors 30
Peripheral resistance 30, 31
Pes planus 319
Physical fitness 225
Physical relaxation 308
Physical therapist 262
    position of 289
Physical therapy 13, 63, 87, 89, 120-122, 124, 131, 132, 147, 202, 230
    evaluation 87
    goals of 63
    intervention 63, 218, 221
    management 10, 12, 48, 69, 77, 87, 124, 126, 134, 135, 137, 222, 225, 227
    plan of 13, 87, 89, 120-122, 124, 131, 132, 147, 202, 230
    postoperative 88
    program, phases of 88, 131
    treatment 46, 161, 168, 217
Physiological relaxation 310
Physiology 28
Physiotherapy 124
Pigeon
    breast 13
    chest 8, 13
Plantar flexion 329
Plethoric appearance 54
Pleura, layers of 1
Pleural cavity 1

Index

Pleural drainage tubes, connection of 192
Pleural effusion 2, 183
Pleural space 193
Pleurisy 2
Pleuropneumonectomy 190
Pneumonectomy 177, 189
   extra-pleural 189
   simple 189
Pneumonia 183
Pneumothorax 2, 127, 150, 184
   chronic 130
   closed 128
Positive expiratory pressure 37, 228
   high pressure 37
   low pressure 37
Positive pressure 194
   breathing, intermittent 298
   oscillating expiratory 228
Postcardiotomy syndrome 184
Posterior basal
   breathing 278
   segment 290*f*
Postoperative complications 180
Postsurgical physical therapy intervention 202
Postural deformity 187, 318
Postural drainage 36, 221, 283
   uses of 36
Postural scoliosis 16
   management of 17
Postural syncope 71
Posture
   bad 317
   dynamic 317
   factors affecting 317
   good 317
   static 317
   types 317
Pott's disease 159
   systemic involvement 160
Pott's paraplegia 159
Pott's spine 159
Power breathe 23
Power lung 23
Practicing relaxation 308
Pregnancy 147
Premature contraction 65
Preoperative pulmonary rehabilitation 200

Preoperative radiotherapy 175
Preoperative surgical physical therapy 88
Pressure resistance 23
Progressive muscle relaxation 308
   technique 309
Proximal muscle pain 12
Pulmonary angiography 166
Pulmonary care 192
Pulmonary contusion 125
Pulmonary edema 53, 306
Pulmonary embolism 140, 184
Pulmonary function
   assessment 50
   measurement of 59, 262
   tests 56, 260, 262
Pulmonary laceration 137, 150
Pulmonary patient, assessment of 50
Pulmonary rehabilitation 199, 256
   assessment for 259
   phases of 200
   postoperative 202
   program 89, 121, 131, 157, 162-164, 168, 267
   treatment of 258
Pulmonary tissue 39
Pulmonary trunk 140, 143
Pulse 81, 110
   altered 114
   oximeter 95, 101
   pressure 32
Pyrexia 114

Q

QRS complex 305
QT syndrome, long 68
Quantitative perfusion 61, 265
Queens step protocol 250

R

Rachitic rosary 11
Radial pulse 9
Radiograph 123, 158, 227
Radiotherapy 174
   postoperative 175
Range of motion 198
Recurrent disease 159
Reflux 71

Relaxation
  advantages of 311
  steps for 308
  techniques 308-310
  types of 308
Relaxed sitting 314f
Renal complications 188
Repolarization 73
Residual volume 57, 60, 61
Respiration 6, 22, 28, 306, 331
  control of 28
  paradoxical 125
Respiratory arrest 185, 302, 331
Respiratory care 267
Respiratory center 28
  function of 28
Respiratory distress 185
  syndrome 307
Respiratory insufficiency, chronic 306
Respiratory movements 20
Respiratory muscle 23, 307
  fatigue 23
  training 23
Respiratory system 331
Respirometer 59, 263
Resting membrane potential 72
Reverse plank bridge 317
Rib 5
  erosion of 173
  false 5
  floating 5
  fracture 123
  resection 155
  true 5
Rickets 8, 11
Right lung, middle lobes of 289
Rotahaler 295
Rotator cuff 326

S

Scalene syndrome 144
Scapula 323
Scheuermann disease 319
Scoliosis 8, 15, 319
  congenital 17
  idiopathic 16
  nonstructural 16
  paralytic 16
  structural 16

Segmentectomy 188
Self drainage 228
Self-bilateral costal expansion 278f
Shaking 36, 269, 270f
Shock 332
  cardiogenic 186
  electric 302
Shoulder
  abduction of 324, 325
  adduction of 324, 325
  exercises 324
  extension of 324
  flexion of 324
  girdle
    depression of 323
    elevation of 323
    exercises 322
    protraction of 323
    retraction of 323, 324
  joint 322
  left 309
  right 309
Side lean standing 316
Sinoatrial node 26
Sinus
  arrhythmia 66
  bradycardia 66
  neat alteration 68
  tachycardia 66
  venosus defect 91
Situational syncope 71
Six-minute walk 61, 265
Skin color, alteration of 114
Small arterioles, caliber of 31
Sneeze 332
Sodium bicarbonate 303
Sounds
  added 55
  voice 55
Speed of paper 73
Sphygmomanometer 332
Spinal curves, functions of 15
Spinal decompression 161
Spinal fusion 161
Spirogram 59, 263
Spirometer 59, 262
Spontaneous pneumothorax 129, 133
Sputum 53, 166
  culture 227
  disposal 301

Index

Squatting 100
Stair climbing 61, 265
Staphylococcus 227
Static compliance 39
Status asthmaticus 224
Stenosis
    aortic 80, 91, 109
    pulmonary 91, 97
    subvalvular 80
    supravalvular 80
    valvular 80
Step test 251
Sternocostal surface 24
Stimulus 34
Strengthening, devices for 23
Stress testing 118
    cardiovascular 63
    thallium 118
Stroke 66, 92
ST-segment elevation myocardial infarction 211
Subcutaneous emphysema 185
Suction 205
    equipment 206
    technique 206
    tubing 206
Supported forward leaning 313, 313*f*
Supportive devices 199
Surgery 101, 135, 212
    contraindications for 84
Surgical physical therapy management 88, 130
Sympathetic nerve supply 26
Syncope 65, 100
    management 70
Syringomyelia 10

T

Tachycardia 65, 239, 332
    atrial paroxysmal 67
    nonsustained ventricular 69
    paroxysmal 67
    supraventricular 68
    ventricular 69
        paroxysmal 68
Tension pneumothorax 129
Tet spells 100
Tetralogy of Fallot 91, 99
Therapeutic relaxation 310

Thoracic aorta injury, descending 142
Thoracic cage 4, 5, 177, 304
    musculature 177
Thoracic incisions 177
Thoracic inlet syndrome 7
Thoracic outlet 144
    vascular injury 141, 144
Thoracic outlet syndrome 144
    arterial 146
    disputed 146
    neurogenic 146
    non-specific 146
    physical therapy management for 147
    types of 144
    vascular 144
    venous 146
Thoracic surgery 123, 177
Thoracotomy 166, 178, 197, 332
    anterior 178
    anterolateral 178
    lateral 178
    posterolateral 179
    tube 135
Thorax 4, 6
    arterial supply of 7
    boundaries of 6
    diaphragm of inlet of 6
    movements 20
    nervous supply of 7
    outlet of 7
    shape of 5
    superior aperture of 6
    venous supply of 7
Throat 310
Thrombosis 332
Thrombus 332
Tidal volume 43, 57, 260
TLCO testing 61
Total lung capacity 57
Trachea 206, 332
    suction 206
Tracheostomy 190, 203
    tube
        functions of 203
        removal of 208
Transabdominal route 304
Transcutaneous electrical nerve stimulation 161

Transthoracic approach 304
Trauma 142
   sonography for 151
Traumatic pneumothorax 128
Treadmill walking test, single-stage 248
Trunk
   cavities 4
   exercises 327
   extension 327
   flexion 327
Tuberculin test 158
Tuberculoma 162
Tuberculosis 164
   active 157, 159
   extrapulmonary 158
   latent 157, 159
   pulmonary 157, 158
   spondylitis 159
   types of 158
Twelve-minute swimming test 251

U

Ultrabreathe 23
Unipolar leads 75
Upper limb muscle, contraction of 269

V

Valve transplant 232
Valvotomy 80, 107
   closed 80
Valvular lesions 78, 105
Vascular abnormalities 166
Vascular symptoms, pathology of 9
Vasodepression syncope 71
Vein 141, 332
Vena caval opening 8
Venous drainage 1, 3
Venous supply 25
Ventilation 41, 43, 46, 196
   artificial 306
   modes of 195
   scanning 61
Ventilator 194
   assisted
      controlled 195
      mechanical 195
   classification of 196
   intermittent mandatory 195
   inverse ratio 195
   muscle
      training 280
      types of 281
   pressure
      ratio mandatory 195
      support 195
   pressure-cycled 196
   setting up 196
   synchronized mandatory 195
   types of 194
   volume-cycled 196
Ventricular extrasystole 67
Ventricular fibrillation 68, 69
Ventricular septal defect 91, 93, 99
Vibration 269f, 285
Viscid mucus 228
Vital capacity 57, 260

W

Waddling gait 12
Wait test 251
Walking test 251
Weaning 206
Weight loss 49
Weight training 49
Wenckebach block 67
Wheeze 332
Wolff-Parkinson-White syndrome 68
Wound complications 187
Wrist
   exercises 326
   extension 326
   flexion 326

EU GSPR Authorised Reprsentative
Logos Europe, 9 rue Nicolas Poussin
1700, La Rochelle, France
Phone: +33 (0) 6 67 93 73 78
E-mail: contact@logoseurope.eu

www.ingramcontent.com/pod-product-compliance
Ingram Content Group UK Ltd.
Pitfield, Milton Keynes, MK11 3LW, UK
UKHW021832140426
5217IPUK00021B/1405